OXFORD MEDICAL PUBLICATIONS

Emergencies
in Psychiatry

Published and forthcoming titles in the Emergencies series:

Emergencies In Anaesthesia
Edited by Keith Allman, Andrew McIndoe, and Iain H. Wilson

Emergencies in Cardiology
Edited by Saul G. Myerson, Robin P. Choudhury, and Andrew Mitchell

Emergencies in Clinical Surgery
Edited by Chris Callaghan, Chris Watson and Andrew Bradley

Emergencies in Critical Care
Edited by Martin Beed, Richard Sherman, and Ravi Mahajan

Emergencies in Nursing
Edited by Philip Downing

Emergencies in Obstetrics and Gynaecology
Edited by S. Arulkumaran

Emergencies in Oncology
Edited by Martin Scott-Brown, Roy A.J. Spence, and Patrick G. Johnston

Emergencies in Paediatrics and Neonatology
Edited by Stuart Crisp and Jo Rainbow

Emergencies in Palliative and Supportive Care
Edited by David Currow and Katherine Clark

Emergencies in Primary Care
Chantal Simon, Karen O'Reilly, John Buckmaster, and Robin Proctor

Emergencies in Psychiatry
Basant K. Puri and Ian H. Treasaden

Emergencies in Radiology
Edited by Richard Graham and Ferdia Gallagher

Emergencies in Respiratory Medicine
Edited by Robert Parker, Catherine Thomas, and Lesley Bennett

Head, Neck and Dental Emergencies
Edited by Mike Perry

Medical Emergencies in Dentistry
Nigel Robb and Jason Leitch

Emergencies in Psychiatry

Basant K. Puri
Professor and Honorary
Consultant in Psychiatry and Imaging
Hammersmith Hospital and
Imperial College London, UK

and

Ian H. Treasaden
Consultant Forensic Psychiatrist
West London Mental Health NHS Trust, UK

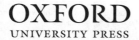

OXFORD
UNIVERSITY PRESS

OXFORD

UNIVERSITY PRESS

Great Clarendon Street, Oxford OX2 6DP

Oxford University Press is a department of the University of Oxford.
It furthers the University's objective of excellence in research, scholarship,
and education by publishing worldwide in

Oxford New York

Auckland Cape Town Dar es Salaam Hong Kong Karachi
Kuala Lumpur Madrid Melbourne Mexico City Nairobi
New Delhi Shanghai Taipei Toronto

With offices in

Argentina Austria Brazil Chile Czech Republic France Greece
Guatemala Hungary Italy Japan Poland Portugal Singapore
South Korea Switzerland Thailand Turkey Ukraine Vietnam

Oxford is a registered trade mark of Oxford University Press
in the UK and in certain other countries

Published in the United States
by Oxford University Press Inc., New York

© Oxford University Press, 2008

British Library Cataloguing in Publication Data

Data available

Library of Congress Cataloging in Publication Data

Data available

Typeset by Newgen Imaging Systems (P) Ltd., Chennai, India
Printed in China
on acid-free paper through
Asia Pacific Offset

ISBN 978–0–19–853080–0 (flexicover: alk.paper)

10 9 8 7 6 5 4 3 2 1

Preface

This is a practical, portable, pocketbook guide to dealing with emergencies in psychiatry.

It is a misconception to believe there are no real true emergencies in psychiatry. In addition, as a practising medical practitioner it is each doctor's responsibility in any case to keep up to date with basic resuscitation procedures and relevant local hospital policies.

Of paramount importance in psychiatric emergencies are the following:

- Ensure your own and staff and, indeed, the patients' safety.
- Always consider an organic causation and try to eliminate this as a potential cause.
- Patient confidentiality is not absolute. The GMC accepts that doctors can reveal information if there is an immediate grave risk to the patient or others ('risk of death or serious harm').
- Always seek corroborative information, e.g. previous medical records, third-party information.
- Consult senior colleagues and/or other members of a multidisciplinary team, including sharing responsibility for difficult decisions.
- Maintain good contemporaneous records of decisions.
- 'If it's not recorded, it didn't happen' is a good precautionary principle. At the least, records are evidence of what may have happened, but in reviews, inquiries and, indeed, in court, doctors will always have the opportunity to expand on their records.

When interviewing patients in situations of psychiatric emergencies, always start initially with open questions, be honest and non-judgemental, and try to direct patients and others away from negative responses towards you. Only make commitments you can keep and that will be acceptable to other members of the multidisciplinary team.

BP
IT
London & Cambridge

Contents

Detailed contents *ix*

Symbols and abbreviations *xix*

1 The assessment of psychiatric emergencies 1
2 The management of psychiatric and medical emergencies 15
3 Psychiatric symptoms and syndromes presenting as emergencies 51
4 Aggression and violence 67
5 Victims of abuse, violence, and disaster 87
6 Homelessness, loneliness, and isolation 109
7 Deliberate self-harm and suicide 115
8 Alcohol misuse and dependence 137
9 Other psychoactive substance misuse 149
10 Emergencies related to psychotropic drug actions 173
11 Psychiatric emergencies in accident and emergency departments 183
12 Psychiatric emergencies in general hospital medical wards 191
13 Psychiatric emergencies in surgical, radiotherapy, oncology, and terminally ill patients 215
14 Psychiatric emergencies in obstetrics and gynaecology 227

15 Psychiatric emergencies in children and
    adolescents   249

16 Psychiatric emergencies in people with
    learning disabilities   259

17 Emergencies in old-age psychiatry   263

18 Emergencies in psychiatry in primary care   273

19 Assertive outreach, crisis resolution and
    intensive home treatment teams, and early
    intervention services   283

20 Mental health legislation relevant to
    emergencies in psychiatry   293

21 Difficult patients and difficult situations   309

22 Emergencies in forensic psychiatry   319

    Index 331

Detailed contents

1   The assessment of psychiatric emergencies   1
    Emergency referrals 2
    Telephone referrals 3
    Interview arrangements 4
    Sources of information 5
    Major emergencies 5
    The interview process 6
    Mental state examination 8
    Mini-Mental State Examination (MMSE) 10
    Physical examination 12
    Investigations 13
    Telepsychiatry 14

2   The management of psychiatric and   15
    medical emergencies
    Emergency interventions 16
    Delirium 18
    General dystonic reactions 22
    Oculogyric crisis 24
    Neuroleptic malignant syndrome 26
    Poisoning 28
    Resuscitation 34
    Wernicke's encephalopathy 42
    Acute severe asthma 45
    Diabetic ketoacidosis and other diabetic
        emergencies 46
    Notifiable diseases 48

Needlestick injuries 49
Human bite wounds 49

3 **Psychiatric symptoms and syndromes presenting**   51
   as emergencies
   Acute psychoses 52
   Endocrinopathies 56
   Disorders presenting with anxiety and panic 58
   Depressive and dysphoric symptomatology 62
   Catatonic patients 64

4 **Aggression and violence**   67
   Schizophrenia and violence 70
   Warning signs 70
   Terminology 70
   Checklist to aid assessment and management 71
   Risk of violence among psychiatric inpatients 72
   Assessment 74
   Risk factors for violence have been recently
       usefully summarized 75
   Management 77
   Summary of management of aggression and
       violence 82
   Safety in outpatient settings 84
   Safety in the community 85
   Burns 86

5 **Victims of abuse, violence, and disaster**   87
   Non-accidental injury of children 88
   Consequences for adult functioning of
       childhood sexual abuse 89
   Child abduction 89
   Spouse abuse (replaces term wife-battering)/
       intimate partner violence 90

Elder abuse *92*

Morbid jealousy (Othello syndrome) *94*

Erotomania (de Clérambault's syndrome) *96*

Stalking *96*

Rape and sexual assault of women *98*

Rape and sexual assault of men *100*

Post-traumatic stress disorder *102*

Acute stress reaction *108*

Adjustment disorder *108*

6   **Homelessness, loneliness, and isolation**   **109**

Prevalence and factors associated with
    homelessness *110*

Housing and mental health *110*

Loneliness *111*

Psychiatric disorders in homeless people *111*

Management of homelessness *112*

Legal framework of management *113*

7   **Deliberate self-harm and suicide**   **115**

Deliberate self-harm *116*

Risk factors for suicide have been recently
    usefully summarized *118*

Assessment of suicidal intent and risk
    of repetition *119*

Management/prognosis/prevention of non-fatal
    deliberate self-harm *119*

Association of suicide with psychiatric
    disorders *120*

Association of suicide with physical disorders *121*

Association with psychiatric hospitalization *122*

Association with general practice consultation *123*

National Confidential Enquiry into Suicide and
        Homicide in the UK 121

Association with antidepressant therapy 128

Referral pathways 131

Assessment and management 132

Discharge 135

Emergency assessment of capacity 136

8   Alcohol misuse and dependence   137
    Units of alcohol 138
    Levels of consumption 139
    Alcohol-related disabilities 140
    Alcohol dependence 142
    Assessment 144
    Acute intoxication 146
    Alcohol withdrawal 147

9   Other psychoactive substance misuse   149
    Misuse of Drugs Act 1971 150
    Opioids 152
    Management of opiate withdrawal 154
    Cannabinoids 156
    Sedatives and hypnotics 158
    Cocaine 160
    Amphetamine and related substances 162
    Caffeine 164
    Hallucinogens 166
    Volatile solvents 170
    History-taking relevant to substance abuse 171
    On examination 171
    Referral to specialist substance misuse
        services 172

Investigations 171
Referral to medical services 172

10 **Emergencies related to psychotropic drug actions**   173
Acute dystonia 174
Clozapine 175
Serotonin syndrome 176
Hyponatraemia and antidepressants 176
Monoamine oxidase inhibitors (MAOIs) 178
Lithium toxicity 181
Paradoxical reactions to benzodiazepines 181

11 **Psychiatric emergencies in accident and**   183
emergency departments
Munchausen syndrome (hospital addiction
   syndrome) 186
Medically unexplained symptoms 188

12 **Psychiatric emergencies in general hospital**   191
medical wards
Epidemiology 192
Prevention 192
Common emergencies in psychiatry in general
   hospital wards 192
Acute organic mental disorder/acute confusional
   states/delirium 194
Memory disturbance 196
Mood disorder 197
Psychiatric aspects of neurology 198
Psychiatric aspects of epilepsy 200
Huntington's disease (chorea) 200
Cerebral tumours 200

Parkinsonism *201*

Multiple sclerosis *201*

Neurosyphilis *201*

HIV/AIDS *201*

Meningitis, encephalitis, and subarachnoid haemorrhages *201*

Psychological reactions to neurological symptoms *201*

Interaction between psychiatric and physical illness *202*

Dissociative and conversion disorders *204*

Hypochondriacal disorder (health anxiety disorder) *204*

Somatization disorder *206*

Medically unexplained symptoms *208*

Factors influencing response to physical illness *208*

Management *209*

Body dysmorphic disorder and other associated concepts *210*

The uncooperative patient *212*

Assessment *212*

Problem of patients taking leave against medical advice before assessment or treatment is complete *213*

13 **Psychiatric emergencies in surgical, radiotherapy, oncology, and terminally ill patients**   **215**

Psychological consequences of surgery *216*

Management of the dying *220*

Bereavement *222*

Atypical (abnormal) complicated grief *224*

14 Psychiatric emergencies in obstetrics and   **227**
    gynaecology

Perinatal psychiatry 228

Post-partum maternity 'blues' 230

Postnatal puerperal depression 232

Puerperal psychosis 236

Role of psychiatric trainee in initial assessment of
    a puerperal woman 239

Other potentially urgent situations relating to
    pregnancy and childbirth 240

Specialist issues to be considered 244

15 Psychiatric emergencies in children   **249**
    and adolescents

Assessment 250

Children Act 1989 251

Safety issues 251

Self-harm 252

Child abuse 254

Other psychiatric emergencies 256

16 Psychiatric emergencies in people with   **259**
    learning disabilities

Presentation 260

Common medical problems 260

Other potential problems 260

Management 261

17 Emergencies in old-age psychiatry   **263**

Presentation of psychiatric disorders 264

Accident and emergency departments 266

Medication 268

Discharge from accident and emergency
departments 271

General management issues in old-age
psychiatry 272

Driving 272

18 Emergencies in psychiatry in primary care 273

Epidemiology 274

Range of cases seen in primary care compared to
psychiatric practice 275

Neurotic and stress-related disorders 276

Safety considerations 282

19 Assertive outreach, crisis resolution and 283
intensive home treatment teams, and early
intervention services

Assertive outreach 285

Crisis resolution and intensive home treatment
teams 288

Early intervention services 290

20 Mental health legislation relevant to 293
emergencies in psychiatry

Mental Health Act 1983 (England and Wales) 294

Definition of categories of mental disorder
recognized in the Mental Health Act 1983 296

Orders under the Mental Health Act 1983 301

Mental Health Review Tribunals (MHRT) 301

Mental Health Act Commission (MHAC)
(Section 121) 302

Court of Protection (Section 94) 302

Patients' rights under Mental Health Act 1983 303

Consent to treatment *303*

Detention under the Mental Health Act on a
general medical or surgical ward *304*

Changes to Mental Health Act 1983 introduced by
Mental Health Act 2006 *305*

Mental Capacity Act 2005 *306*

Assessment of capacity under the Mental Capacity
Act 2005 *306*

Provisions of Mental Capacity Act 2005 *306*

Mental Capacity Act 2005 *307*

Code of practice for Mental Capacity Act 2005 *308*

21 **Difficult patients and difficult situations** 309

Psychodynamic aspects of the management of
psychiatric emergencies *310*

Managing difficult patients *312*

Understanding the psychodynamics of being
mentally disordered *314*

Particular situations of difficulty *316*

22 **Emergencies in forensic psychiatry** 319

Police and court liaison *320*

Psychiatric expert evidence for court *324*

Problem areas in police/court liaison and
reporting *326*

Prison psychiatry *328*

Index *331*

Symbols and abbreviations

ABG	arterial blood gases
AUDIT	Alcohol Use Disorders Identification Test
CAMHS	Child and Adolescent Mental Health Service
EPDS	Edinburgh Postnatal Depression Scale
FAS	fetal alcohol syndrome
FAST	Fast Alcohol Screening Test
FBC	full blood count
GAF	Global Assessment of Functioning
GGT	gamma glutamyl transpeptidase
HAV	hepatitis A virus
HBV	hepatitis B virus
HCV	hepatitis C virus
IUCD	intrauterine contraceptive device
IM	intramuscular/ly
INR	international normalized ratio (prothrombin ratio)
IV	intravenous/ly
LFT	liver function test
LSD	lysergic acid diethylamine
MAOI	monoamine oxidase inhibitor
MCV	mean corpuscular volumes
MDE	major depressive episode
MDMA	3,4-methylenedioxy-N-methylamphetamine
MHAC	Mental Health Act Commission
MHRT	Mental Health Review Tribunal
MMSE	Mini-Mental State Examination
PMS	premenstrual tension syndrome
SADQ	Severity of Alcohol Dependence Questionnaire
SSRI	selective serotonin reuptake inhibitor
U&E	urea and electrolytes & creatinine in plasma

The assessment of psychiatric emergencies

Emergency referrals 2
Telephone referrals 3
Interview arrangements 4
Sources of information 5
Major emergencies 5
The interview process 6
Mental state examination 8
Mini-Mental State Examination (MMSE) 10
Physical examination 12
Investigations 13
Telepsychiatry 14

:⚙: Emergency referrals

Emergency referrals in psychiatry form a significant percentage of clinical work while on call and can reflect the interface between routine psychiatric casework and the wider context in which the clinician practises.

Soon after starting work in psychiatry, it becomes clear that these types of referrals can come from a variety of sources. Many are from hospital doctors. Different types of referral from various medical and surgical specialities are covered in later chapters of this book, particularly Chapters 12–14. Psychiatric emergencies presenting to accident and emergency departments are another important source of referrals, and are considered in more detail in Chapter 11. Psychiatric emergencies related to primary care are discussed in Chapter 18.

A common means by which emergency psychiatric referrals are made is via the telephone. In this chapter an account is given of the key points to bear in mind in relation to such telephone referrals. This is followed by a consideration of interview arrangements, sources of information, and the psychiatric assessment. Finally, a brief description is also given of the newly emerging field of telepsychiatry.

ⓘ Telephone referrals

Adopting a systematic approach allows the following important information to be garnered in an efficient manner during a telephone referral of an emergency psychiatry case:

- Details of the person making the referral
  - Their name
  - Contact details
  - Relationship to the patient (e.g. general practitioner or social worker)
- How urgent is the referral?
- Details of the patient being referred
  - Name
  - Date of birth
  - Address
  - Current location
  - Legal status (with respect to the Mental Health Act or equivalent legislation)
  - Telephone number
  - Hospital number
  - Name and address of general practitioner
  - Name of hospital (and, if possible, consultant) at which they have previously received psychiatric care
- Major complaint
  - Nature of the complaint
  - History of the present illness
- Primary requirement of the person making the referral
  - Would they like you to assess the case with a view to an emergency inpatient admission?
  - Would they like a domiciliary visit?
  - Would advice over the telephone suffice?
  - Would they like an outpatient appointment to be made?
- Substance misuse history
- Any relevant forensic history
- Any specific areas of risk, e.g. violence
- Current treatment and any known allergies
- Past medical history
- Any other information which the person making the referral feels you need to know.

Patient confidentiality should be ensured at all times. Do not give out any confidential information during a telephone call to someone you do not know. (Journalists and private detectives could conceivably pose as doctors to try to obtain sensitive information.)

Interview arrangements

The key aims of the psychiatry interview are[1]:
- To obtain information
- To assess the emotions and attitudes of the patient
- To supply a supportive role and allow an understanding of the patient. This is the basis of the subsequent working relationship with the patient.

It is vitally important to ensure that you are safe during the interview, especially during the psychiatric emergency assessment of a patient you have never met.

As part of your training, it is useful to obtain practical instruction in simple breakaway techniques. The following interview arrangements can help to minimize the risks to your safety[2]:

- Bear in mind that patients who are hostile and angry cannot always be talked down, especially if they are very paranoid, psychotic or have an organic mental disorder.
- If interviewing in a hospital, always tell other members of staff which patient you will be interviewing and where, and be aware of relevant ward policies on violence, as well as alarm systems and bells.
- It may be necessary to alert the hospital security staff that their assistance may be required in the course of an assessment.
- If interviewing in a police station, ensure that the duty officer knows which interview room or police cell you are going to use and whom you will be interviewing. If you are at all concerned, you may ask for a police officer to sit in with you.
- Rapport is increased and the risk of violence diminished if you sit about 1 yard away from the patient, at the same level and in a position from which you can always look at the patient but they can look away. This is usually achieved by sitting at right angles.
- Both you and the patient should have free access to the door (unless the patient is being detained, for example in a police or prison cell). This way, the patient does not feel trapped and you can make an easy exit if need be.
- Should a patient become acutely angry or threatening, you should adopt a calm manner, talk in a quiet voice, avoid eye contact, and sit rather than stand to avoid making the patient feel overwhelmed period. You may need to be prepared to talk a patient down for a prolonged period.
- If carrying out an emergency psychiatric assessment in a patient's home, never agree to do so in a room, such as the kitchen, where potential weapons (such as kitchen knives) may be present.

References

1 Institute of Psychiatry (1973). *Notes on Eliciting and Recording Clinical Information.* Oxford University Press: Oxford.
2 Puri BK, Laking PJ, Treasaden IH (2002). *Textbook of Psychiatry*, 2nd edn. Churchill Livingstone: Edinburgh.

Sources of information

Sources of further information about the patient, which should be consulted, may include the following:

- General practitioner
- Case notes
- Relatives
- Friends and other associates
- Social worker
- Community psychiatric nurse
- Hostel staff.

A request can be made that any discharge summaries from previous admissions to another hospital be faxed to you.

☠ Major emergencies

If you are called to deal with a major emergency, such as someone threatening to jump off a roof or a person threatening others with a weapon, ensure that the appropriate authorities are contacted. These would normally consist of the police in the community and the security personnel in a hospital. (Make sure you know the number for contacting security in an emergency in your hospital.) It is best to liaise with this authority (the police, hospital security, or sometimes the fire service or armed services) and allow them to take overall control.

The interview process

You should take the time to conduct a professional detailed interview process with the patient. Although it is important to take into account corroborative history and tentative diagnoses from other professionals, a clinical diagnosis needs to be arrived at by first interviewing the patient in person. This may help to uncover other aspects of the case such as aetiological factors which may help in the management of the emergency. The interview process involves bringing together information gleaned from other sources (see above) with that obtained directly from the patient. In respect of the latter, the details relating to the following headings of the psychiatric history should be obtained, if possible[1]:

- Reason for referral
- Symptoms/complaints
- History of presenting illness, including onset, triggers, progression
  - Why has the patient presented at this time in this particular way?
- Recent major life events such as bereavement
- Family history
- Family psychiatric history
- Personal history
- Childhood
- Education
- Occupational history
- Psychosexual history
- Children
- Current social situation
- Past medical history, including a history of head injuries and epilepsy
- Past psychiatric history, including episodes of self-harm
- Psychoactive substance use
  - Alcohol—including the FAST and CAGE questionnaires
  - Tobacco
  - Illicit drug abuse
- Forensic history
- Premorbid personality.

Reference

1 Puri BK, Laking PJ, Treasaden IH (2002). *Textbook of Psychiatry*, 2nd edn. Churchill Livingstone: Edinburgh.

Mental state examination

The main areas which should be covered during the mental state examination, with which the reader is expected to be familiar (see Puri et al., 2002[1] for further details if required), are as follows.

- Appearance and behaviour
  - General appearance
  - Eye contact
  - Facial appearance
- Manner
  - Rapport
  - Anxious
  - Hostile
- Motility
  - Posture, e.g. waxy flexibility
  - Movements
    —mannerisms
    —stereotypes
    —tics
    —orofacial dyskinesias
  - Underactivity
  - Overactivity
- Speech
  - Rate, e.g. fast, under pressure, slow, sudden silences
  - Quantity
  - Articulation
  - Poverty
- Mood
  - Anxiety
  - Sadness
  - Elation
  - Reactive
  - Incongruous
  - Affect
- Thought
  - Form, e.g. flight of ideas, formal schizophrenic thought disorder
  - Content
    —poverty
    —paranoid
    —preoccupations
    —obsessions
    —phobias
    —hypochondriacal
    —pessimistic
    —suicidal thoughts
    —homicidal thoughts

- Abnormal beliefs and interpretations of events
  - Overvalued ideas
  - Delusions (false beliefs), including passivity phenomena (externally controlled)
  - Delusional perception
- Abnormal experiences
  - Sensory distortions—illusions (misperceptions)
  - Sensory deceptions—hallucinations (perceptions in the absence of external stimuli)
  - Disorders of self-awareness
- Cognitive state
  - Orientation
    —day
    —date
    —time
    —place
  - Attention
    —serial sevens (subtraction from 100)
  - Concentration
  - Memory
    —recent, e.g. age, name of prime minister
    —distant, e.g. date of birth, name of sovereign
    —name and address memory test
  - General knowledge
  - Intelligence
  - Formal Mini-Mental State Examination (MMSE).

Insight: this would include an account from the patient of his or her understanding of the factors leading to the current situation as compared to an objective assessment by the clinician. Does the patient consider himself or herself to be ill? If so, physically or mentally ill? Is there insight into particular delusions? Does the patient consider their condition reactive to the situation or occurring out of the blue? Does the patient consider they require outpatient or inpatient psychiatric treatment, including medication? (Note that it is useful to compare the patient's narrative of his illness with an objective evaluation by the examiner.)

In addition to having a pivotal role in the psychiatric diagnostic process, eliciting evidence of certain abnormalities of the mental state, such as the presence of suicidal and/or homicidal thoughts, is clearly of great importance in the assessment of the psychiatric emergency.

Reference

1 Puri BK, Laking PJ, Treasaden IH (2002). *Textbook of Psychiatry*, 2nd edn. Churchill Livingstone: Edinburgh.

Mini-Mental State Examination (MMSE)[1]

The score for a patient is calculated using the following assessments, out of a total maximum score of 30:

1. Orientation in time: the patient is asked to give the year, season, date, month and day of the week. One point is scored for each of these correctly answered. Maximum score is 5.

2. Orientation in place: the patient is asked to give the country, city, part of the city, street and house or flat number (or their equivalent, e.g. name of hospital and name or number of the ward). One point is scored for each of these correctly answered. Maximum score is 5.

3. Registration: name three objects and ask the patient to repeat these immediately. One point is scored for each object correctly named. Maximum score is 3. Then ask the patient to repeat these objects (up to six trials) until they have registered them correctly.

4. Attention and concentration: serial sevens test (see above), stopping after five answers. One point is scored for each correct subtraction by seven. Alternatively, the patient can be asked to spell the word 'WORLD' backwards, in which case the score is the total number of letters which appear in the correct (that is, reverse) order. Maximum score is 5.

5. Recall: the patient is asked to recall the three objects named earlier (see 3). One point is scored for each object correctly named. Maximum score is 3.

6. Language functions: check that the patient is wearing their reading glasses if they need them. The patient is then shown an everyday object (such as a pencil) and asked to name it. They are then shown another everyday object (such as a watch) and again asked to name this. One point is scored for each object correctly named. Maximum score is 2.

7. Language functions: the patient is asked to repeat the following sentence (which is said out loud to the patient): 'No ifs, ands or buts.' One point is scored if this sentence is repeated correctly.

8. The patient is instructed to: 'Take this piece of paper in your right hand, fold it in half, and place it on the floor.' (Or a similar command.) There are three parts to this command, and one point is scored for each part correctly performed. Maximum score is 3.

9. On the reverse side of a sheet of paper, print the words 'CLOSE YOUR EYES' in large enough letters for the patient. The patient is told that they are about to be shown an instruction, which they should read and follow (after putting on their reading glasses should they need them). One point is scored if the patient correctly closes their eyes after reading the instruction.

10. Ask the patient to write a sentence. One point is scored if the patient writes down a sensible sentence which contains a subject and a verb.
11. The patient is shown a design consisting of two intersecting pentagons, such as that shown below. One point is scored if this is copied correctly (with no deduction for a change in rotation of the whole picture or the effects of tremor).

A total MMSE score of no greater than 24 is generally taken as indicative of dementia, in the absence of delirium, schizophrenia or a severe depressive state.

Reference

1 Folstein MF, Folstein SE, McPugh PR (1975). 'Mini-mental state'. A practical method for grading the cognitive state of patients for the clinician. *Journal of Psychiatric Research* **12**: 189–98.

Physical examination

There appears to be an increasing trend these days for psychiatric patients not to be given a full physical examination. It is the view of the authors that this is a mistake. It is easy to miss many organic pathologies by not carrying out a detailed physical examination. Furthermore, certain physical findings may have an important bearing on the choice of medication, as well as potentially revealing side-effects of current or recent treatment. As the reader is expected to be medically qualified, details of how to carry out a physical examination are not given here.

Finer detail should be needs-based and led by relevant findings. If you suspect that the patient may be suffering from an organic cerebral disorder, then some or all of the following cerebral functions should be checked:

- Check the level of consciousness (from fully awake, through drowsiness, stuporose, semi-comatose to deep coma (and then death))
- Check for clouding of consciousness, delirium and fugue
- Check for evidence of an oneiroid (dreamlike) state, twilight state and torpor
- Language ability
- Check for dysarthrias, paraphasias, neologisms, telegraphic speech and aphasias
- Handedness
- Non-verbal memory
- Apraxia
  - Check for constructional apraxia, visuospatial agnosia, dressing apraxia, ideomotor apraxia and ideational apraxia
- Agnosias and disorders of body image
  - Check for visual (object) agnosia, prosopagnosia, agnosia for colours, simultagnosia, agraphognosia (agraphaesthesia), anosognosia, coenestopathic states, autotopagnosia, astereognosia, finger agnosia, topographical disorientation, distorted awareness of size and shape, hemisomatognosia (hemidepersonalization) and the reduplication phenomenon
- Number functions
- Right–left disorientation
- Verbal fluency
- Abstraction
- Similarities
- Alternating sequences
- Motor sequencing.

Investigations

Depending on your differential diagnosis, it may be appropriate to request or carry out further investigations, such as:

- Blood tests, e.g. full blood count, urea and electrolytes, thyroid function tests, liver function tests, syphilitic serology, lithium level
- Illicit drug screen (urinary or salivary screen for illicit drugs)
- Electroencephalography, e.g. if epilepsy is suspected
- Neuropsychological tests, e.g. if dementia or pseudodementia is suspected
- Neuroimaging, e.g. to exclude a brain tumour, cerebral secondaries or multiple sclerosis, or to check for cortical atrophy or a haematoma.

☠ Telepsychiatry

As far back as the 1970s, the potential role of telecommunications in making psychiatric assessments was predicted[1]:

> 'Because technological innovations will enable geographic proximity to be replaced eventually by electronic proximity, telecommunication systems could play a substantial role in psychiatry's future.'

Telepsychiatry is beginning to be used in psychiatry emergency assessments. For example, a multispecialty telephone and e-mail consultation service is available for patients with developmental disabilities in rural California. Consultations for psychiatry form a key service request. They were found to have constituted 10 out of the first 30 consultations, all by telephone, as follows[2]:

Table 1.1

Consultation type	Number of patients
Agitation ± aggression	5
Agitation/sexual behaviour	1
Aggression/insomnia	1
Depression	1
Insomnia	1
Bipolar disorder	1

Each telephone consultation lasted between 30 minutes and 1 hour.

A Finnish follow-up study of 60 consecutive patients referred to an acute open ward after having their first psychiatric contact through a video link with the psychiatrist on duty[3] concluded that there were only minor technical problems and that:

> 'The results suggest both acceptance and satisfaction on the part of patients and staff with new technology, instead of waiting for a consultation or traveling to see a psychiatrist in a face-to-face meeting. Telepsychiatry seems to be suitable for the assessment of psychiatric emergency patients, and satisfactory for patients and staff alike.'

References

1 Maxmen JS (1978). Telecommunications in psychiatry. *American Journal of Psychotherapy* **32**: 450–6.
2 Hilty DM, Ingraham RL, Yang SP, Anders TF (2004). Multispecialty telephone and e-mail consultation for patients with developmental disabilities in rural California. *Telemedicine Journal and e-Health* **10**: 413–21.
3 Sorvaniemi M, Ojanen I, Santamäki O (2005). Telepsychiatry in emergency consultations: a follow-up study of sixty patients. *Telemedicine Journal and e-Health* **11**: 439–41.

The management of psychiatric and medical emergencies

Emergency interventions 16
Delirium 18
General dystonic reactions 22
Oculogyric crisis 24
Neuroleptic malignant syndrome 26
Poisoning 28
Resuscitation 34
Wernicke's encephalopathy 42
Acute severe asthma 45
Diabetic ketoacidosis and other diabetic emergencies 46
Notifiable diseases 48
Needlestick injuries 49
Human bite wounds 49

Emergency interventions

This chapter deals with the following clinical emergencies which the psychiatrist may have to diagnose and manage in the first instance: delirium, oculogyric crisis, neuroleptic malignant syndrome, drug poisoning, resuscitation, Wernicke's encephalopathy, acute severe asthma, diabetic ketoacidosis, hypoglycaemia in insulin-dependent diabetes mellitus, notifiable diseases, infectious diseases, needle-stick injuries, and bite injuries. In each case, it is important to be able to assess the urgency of case and the requirement for admission to a medical (or psychiatric) ward correctly, if the patient is not presently an inpatient. Liaison with staff from medical firms is clearly important, and appropriate follow-up arrangements must be made once the emergency intervention has been successful.

☀ Delirium

Clinical features

This may be the most common psychiatric disorder encountered by trainees and medical students in hospital non-psychiatric wards. Calls to psychiatrists often come at dusk when the loss of daylight precipitates symptoms. Delirium is characterized by acute generalized psychological dysfunction which usually fluctuates in degree and which involves impairment of consciousness and attention, with the level of consciousness being between full wakefulness and stupor (see Fig. 2.1). It tends to develop over a relatively short period, of hours to days. Delirium is often accompanied by disturbances in:

- Perception, particularly in the visual modality—illusions, hallucinations, metamorphosias
- Mood—anxiety, lability or depressed mood
- Psychomotor behaviour—hyperactivity, hypoactivity
- Circadian rhythm
- Thoughts—including delusions (often paranoid)
- Memory—particularly impairment of immediate recall and recent memory
- Orientation—particularly temporal disorientation.
  Prodromal symptoms include:
- Confusion/perplexity
- Agitation
- Hypersensitivity to light and sound.

Differential diagnosis

The most important differential diagnoses for delirium are:
Dementia. With the important exception of dementia caused by some cerebrovascular accidents, the onset of dementia is usually insidious. Dementia is often progressive and does not adversely affect the level of consciousness until late in the illness. Although poor memory is a feature of both delirium and dementia, inattention is uncommon in dementia, at least in its early stages. Comorbidity of dementia and delirium is relatively common, particularly in elderly patients.

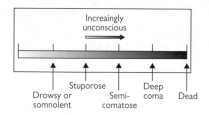

Fig. 2.1 The Spectrum of conscious level, showing the position of delirium.

- *Depressive episodes*. The level of consciousness is usually not impaired in depression, while clinical symptomatology may show diurnal variation. The memory is generally unaffected. If they occur, hallucinations in depression tend to be in the auditory modality, while delusions, if they occur, tend to be mood-congruent and generally not as fragmented or short-lived as in delirium. Clinically, it is important to take hydration/nutritional status of a severely depressed patient into account when thinking about diagnosis and management of risk.
- *Schizophrenia*. The level of consciousness in schizophrenia is usually not impaired, although in acute schizophrenia the patient may appear perplexed. While attention may be impaired, the memory is generally not as overtly affected as it is in delirium. If they occur, hallucinations tend to be in the auditory modality in schizophrenia. The delusions of schizophrenia are generally not as fragmented or short-lived as in delirium.
- *Substance-induced* (withdrawal or intoxication).
- *Drug-induced* (particularly drug interactions in the elderly).

Aetiology

Note that the cause may not be evident at first. Awareness of this will help avoid pointless arguments between psychiatrists and other medical practitioners who may insist that it cannot be delirium because 'we have excluded all causes'. There are many potential causes of delirium, including the following.

Drugs and alcohol
- Toxicity with prescribed drugs, illicit drugs, alcohol, inhalants, industrial poisons (such as organic solvents and heavy metals), and carbon monoxide
- Withdrawal from drugs and alcohol.

Intracranial causes
- Infection—encephalitis, meningitis, abscesses, syphilis, HIV/AIDS
- Head injury
- Subarachnoid haemorrhage
- Brain tumours
- Subdural haematoma
- Transient ischaemic attack
- Cerebral oedema
- Cerebral aneurysm
- Intraparenchymal haemorrhage
- Hypertensive encephalopathy
- Cerebral vasculitis.

Metabolic and endocrine disorders
- Hypoxia
- Hypoglycaemia
- Hyperglycaemia
- Volume depletion
  - Fluid imbalance/hypovolumic states

- Volume overloading
  - Fluid imbalance/hypervolumic states
- Acidosis
- Alkalosis
- Anaemia
- Uraemia
- Vitamin deficiency—thiamine, nicotinic acid, folate, pyridoxine, vitamin B12
- Vitamin excess—vitamin A, vitamin D
- Hypoalbuminaemia
- Hyperalbuminaemia
- Bilirubinaemia
- Raised or lowered plasma levels of calcium, potassium, sodium or magnesium
- Hypophosphataemia
- Errors of metabolism—porphyria
- Addison's disease
- Cushing's syndrome
- Hyperinsulinism
- Hypothyroidism
- Hyperthyroidism
- Hypoparathyroidism
- Hyperparathyroidism
- Hypopituitarism
- Carcinoid syndrome.

Systemic infections
- Bacteraemia
- Sepsis
- Viral infections
- Fungal infections
- Protozoal infections.

Miscellaneous
- Postoperative states
- Seizures
- Epilepsy
- Postictal states
- Neoplasia
- Hypothermia
- Radiation
- Immunosuppression
- Fractures
- Electrocution.

Other central nervous system disorders
- Huntington's disease
- Hydrocephalus
- Multiple sclerosis
- Parkinson's disease
- Wilson's disease.

Organ failure
- Hepatic
- Renal
- Respiratory
- Cardiac
- Pancreatic.

Toxicity with many prescribed drugs
- Analgesics—such as salicylates and opiates
- Antibiotics—including cephalosporins, chloramphenicol, sulphonamides and tetracycline
- Anticonvulsants—including phenobarbital, phenytoin and valproate
- Anti-inflammatory drugs—including corticosteroids, ibuprofen, indomethacin and naproxen
- Antineoplastic agents
- Antiparkinsonian drugs
- Antituberculous drugs
- Antiviral drugs
- Barbiturates
- Benzodiazepines
- Cardiac drugs—including digitalis preparations (digoxin, digitoxin), β-adrenoceptor antagonists and ACE inhibitors
- Chloroquine
- Cimetidine
- Lithium salts
- Phenelzine
- Ranitidine
- Sympathomimetics–e.g. cold cures.

Management

Delirium may have to be managed supportively/symptomatically initially. This involves maintaining stability of the patient's vital functions in the short term. It is important in the medium term to work towards the underlying cause(s) of the delirium which should be determined by carrying out any necessary investigations, and this (they) should then be treated. Pending the establishment of the cause(s), supportive medical and symptomatic treatment may be required.

Good, calming nursing is needed, preferably in a quiet single room, with a reality orientation approach, with reorientation by staff and low-level nocturnal lighting, and involving a multidisciplinary team. Ensure that the patient has an adequate fluid and electrolyte balance. The patient should be reassured, and helped to deal with any frightening illusions, hallucinations, and delusions.

If medication is required for agitation or anxiety, then a very low dose of haloperidol (oral or intramuscular) can be used, unless the patient is suffering from hepatic failure, in which case a very low dose of a benzodiazepine may be required instead. Short-acting rather than long-acting drugs are to be preferred in this context. A second low dose of haloperidol may be administered after 2 h. All medication should be reviewed regularly (at least daily). The exception to this in psychiatry may be the case of substance-induced delirious states.

☻ General dystonic reactions

Dystonia can occur on starting, increasing, or withdrawing antipsychotics, especially older typical antipsychotics. Features of general dystonic reactions include:

- More common in young men (related to muscle mass)
- Seen in approximately 10% of patients exposed to older typical drugs (phenothiazines, butyrophenones)[1]. Main features are torticollis, oculogyric crisis, tongue protrusion, grimacing, and opisthotonos
- Patients may be unable to swallow or speak clearly
- In extreme cases the back may arch or the jaw dislocate
- It can be both painful and very frightening.

📖 Treatment of general dystonic reactions is described on p. 80.

Reference

1 American Psychiatric Association (1997). Practice guideline for the treatment of patients with schizophrenia. American Psychiatric Association. *American Journal of Psychiatry* **154**: 1–63.

☀ Oculogyric crisis

Clinical features

This is an acute dystonic reaction that is relatively rarely seen nowadays owing to increased use of newer atypical antipsychotics; it is less common than general dystonic reactions. After an initial phase in which the patient may be restless or agitated and during which they might develop a fixed stare, the full-blown oculogyric crisis characteristically manifests with an arched neck and involuntary movement of the eyes superiorly and possibly laterally. Convergence and downward movement of the eyes have also been described. The tongue may be protruded and the mouth opened widely. Rapid blinking, lacrimation, mutism or palilalia (in which a word is repeated with increasing frequency), and tachycardia may also occur.

A recent review by Abe (2006)[1] has reported that both antipsychotic-induced oculogyric crises and postencephalitic oculogyric crises have the following features in common:

• They tend to occur late in the day
• They tend to occur at regular intervals
• Associated autonomic symptoms tend to occur—such as profuse sweating, facial flushing, transitory hypertension and difficulty in micturition
• They are often associated with transient episodes of psychopathology such as visual hallucinations, visual illusions, auditory hallucinations, delusions, catatonic phenomena, obsessive thoughts, and panic attacks.

Aetiology

Most cases seen in psychiatric patients are induced by antipsychotic (both typical and atypical) medication. Other medical causes of oculogyric crisis include:

• Postencephalitic Parkinson's disease
• Herpes encephalitis
• Juvenile Parkinson's disease
• Non-antipsychotic psychotropic drugs—such as benzodiazepines, lithium salts, carbamazepine, tricyclic antidepressants, and reserpine
• Other drugs—such as metoclopramide (which is a substituted benzamide), cisplatin, levodopa, nifedipine, and chloroquine
• Influenza immunization
• Head injury
• Neurosyphilis
• Multiple sclerosis
• Tourette's (Gilles de la Tourette's) syndrome
• Bilateral thalamic infarction
• Cystic glioma of the third ventricle
• Fourth ventricle lesions.

Management

It is important to start by reviewing the current medications and doses received within the past 24 h. If the cause is clearly likely to be antipsychotic medication, then the patient should be reassured, and an antimuscarinic drug such as procyclidine or benzatropine may be administered parenterally. Regular prescription of oral antimuscarinics may be required in the short term, but the ongoing need for this should be regularly reviewed. After dealing with the emergency, consideration should be given to changing the antipsychotic drug which caused the reaction. It is necessary, however, to be aware of manufacturers' guidelines on stopping/switching/titrating antipsychotics and not do this in a cavalier and risky fashion.

If the patient is not taking antipsychotic medication, then the cause needs to be found. This may be clear from the medication that the patient is taking; for example, a patient on an oncology ward may be taking metoclopramide and/or cisplatin. A full history, careful perusal of the case notes, a physical examination and appropriate investigations may be required.

Reference

1 Abe K (2006). Psychiatric symptoms associated with oculogyric crisis: a review of literature for the characterization of antipsychotic-induced episodes. *World Journal of Biological Psychiatry* **7**: 70–4.

☠ Neuroleptic malignant syndrome

This uncommon neuroleptic-induced movement disorder is a medical emergency that is life-threatening and requires immediate treatment. It most often occurs with drugs which act directly on central dopaminergic systems, but has also been reported with other drugs including tricyclic antidepressants. It is likely to be an idiosyncratic reaction and some patients have been cautiously re-challenged with the same agent without recurrence. The Canadian Movement Disorders Group has estimated that 0.5–1% of patients exposed to neuroleptics will develop this syndrome, with most developing it shortly after initial exposure (90% within 2 weeks). High potency typical antipsychotics such as haloperidol are more likely to cause this syndrome.

Clinical features

The clinical features of neuroleptic malignant syndrome include:
- Autonomic dysfunction
  - Hyperthermia
  - Labile blood pressure
  - Pallor
  - Sweating
  - Tachycardia
- Fluctuating level of consciousness (stupor)
- Muscular rigidity
- Urinary incontinence.

Symptoms may last for up to 1 week after cessation of the offending antipsychotic drug; in the case of depot antipsychotic medication, the neuroleptic malignant syndrome may last longer than a week.

Investigations

Blood tests may show:
- Raised serum creatine kinase
- Leukocytosis.

Management

This is a clinical emergency. The causative antipsychotic drug should be stopped immediately. The patient should be admitted as an inpatient to a medical ward where maximal supportive care should be instituted. Sometimes dantrolene or bromocriptine (a dopamine agonist) may be required.

If the same antipsychotic is to be reintroduced, then a period of at least 2 weeks should elapse in the case of oral medication and a period of at least 6 weeks in the case of parenteral medication. The patient should be carefully monitored at this time for any signs of re-emergence of this syndrome. However, it may be more sensible to use a different, low potency, antipsychotic instead of the drug which was associated with the original episode.

Prognosis

There may be complications such as renal failure or respiratory failure. The overall mortality rate is greater than 10%.

:☠: Poisoning

In the UK, advice is available 24 h per day from the UK National Poisons Information Service (Tel. 0870 600 6266 in the UK) and from TOXBASE (via the internet web site www.spib.axl.co.uk). General measures in the treatment of acute poisoning are given in the *Oxford Handbook of Clinical Medicine*[1] and are reproduced here with permission.

Psychiatric assessment

Interview informants, family, and friends.

The following point to intention:
• Planned
• Precautions taken to avoid being found
• Was help sought
• Had the patient considered that he or she had taken sufficient to kill self or be dangerous
• Suicide note
• Active hostility aimed at another.

Present intention:
• Precipitant to self-poisoning
• Still present?

Factors associated with suicide risk:
• Psychiatric disorder, e.g. depression, alcoholism, schizophrenia, personality disorder
• Previous suicide attempts
• Socially isolated without support
• Male, unemployed, over 50 years of age.

Note that the risk of completed suicide is increased in the first year, particularly the first 6 months, following deliberate self-harm. While prediction is difficult, the closer the clinical and demographic characteristics are to completed suicide, the greater the risk. One per cent of patients who deliberately self-harm commit suicide in the first year. Of deliberate self-harm patients, 10% ultimately commit suicide, and 50% of completed suicides have a history of deliberate self-harm.

Refer to psychiatric services, especially if at high suicidal risk, psychiatric disorder. To prevent leaving the accident department or hospital, ward the following can be used:
• Common law
• Detention under the Mental Health Act 1983.

The competency of an individual who is self-poisoning to take his leave against medical advice may always be questioned. Act first and dispute later.

Individual drugs

Table 2.1 Individual drugs

Poison	Key symptoms and signs of poisoning	Initial treatment. Always seek expert help as soon as possible
Benzodiazepines	Respiratory arrest	Flumazenil (which may provoke fits)
β-blockers	Severe bradycardia or hypotension	Atropine. If fails then glucagon bolus + 5% dextrose
Carbon monoxide	Pink/pale skin, headache, vomiting, tachycardia, tachypnoea; fits, coma and cardiac arrest if carboxyhaemoglobin level rises above 50%	• Remove source of CO • 100% oxygen • Mannitol IV if cerebral oedema
Cyanide	Fast-killing (uncouples mitochondrial oxidative phosphorylation)—respiratory arrest, preceded by hyper ventilation, is the primary cause of death	• 100% oxygen • GI decontamination • ± (sodium nitrite + sodium thiosulfate) or (dicobalt edentate IV) or hydroxocobalamin
Ecstasy (MDMA)	May include nausea, myalgia, amnesia, blurred vision, pyrexia, confusion, ataxia, arrhythmias, hyperthermia, acute renal failure, cardiovascular collapse, disseminated intravascular coagulation, and acute respiratory distress syndrome	No specific antidote. Supportive treatment required. Management may include: • Activated charcoal • Diazepam for anxiety • If hyperthermic (with rectal temperature >39°C) (akin to serotonin syndrome) —Attempt to cool —Propranolol, muscle relaxation and ventilation may also be required
Opiates (also contained in many analgesic preparations)	Inadequate respiration	Naloxone IV (may precipitate opiate withdrawal)
Paracetamol	No symptoms or signs initially. Later, signs of hepatic and renal failure develop	Should treat immediately and not wait for hepatocellular necrosis • Lavage within 1 h if >12 g taken or level >150 mg/kg • Activated charcoal if less than 8 h since ingestion

Table 2.1 (Contd.)

Poison	Key symptoms and signs of poisoning	Initial treatment. Always seek expert help as soon as possible
		• If plasma paracetamol concentration above the normal treatment line (see Fig. 2.2) treat with IV infusion of acetylcysteine or, if the overdose was taken within the previous 10–12 h, with oral methionine
		• Malnourished patients (e.g. Those with anorexia, depression, alcoholism, HIV-positive) and/or those on hepatic enzyme inducing drugs (e.g. carbamazepine, alcohol) should be treated as above if their plasma-paracetamol concentration is above the high-risk treatment line (see Fig. 2.2)
Paraquat (in weed killers)	Alveolitis, renal failure, oral ulceration, diarrhoea, and vomiting Urine test diagnostic	Activated charcoal and then a laxative
Organophosphate insecticides	Inactivation of choli nesterase leads to the SLUD response (Salivation, Lacrimation, Urination, and Diarrhoea)	Wear gloves Remove soiled clothes Wash skin Take blood for FBC and serum cholinesterase Atropine IV Contact Poisons Information Service
Salicylate (aspirin and many other over-the-counter remedies)	Early features may include vomiting, dehydration, hyper ventilation, tinnitus, vertigo, and sweating. Respiratory alkalosis and then metabolic acidosis	Correct dehydration If within 1 h of overdose, gastric lavage ± activated charcoal Take paracetamol and salicylate levels, in addition to glucose, U&E, LFTs, INR, ABG, bicarbonate, and FBC If metabolic acidosis, treat with sodium bicarbonate (but note that hypokalaemia may occur; therefore monitor serum K^+)

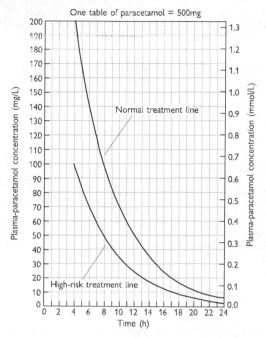

Fig. 2.2 Plasma-paracetamol concentration curves. Reproduced with kind permission from *The British National Formulary* September 2007. For current BNF guidelines please visit BNF.org.

Antidepressants, lithium salts, phenothiazines and related drugs

The 54th edition of the *British National Formulary* (BMJ Publishing Group and RPS Publishing, 2007) gives the following advice, reproduced with permission, for dealing with poisoning with antidepressants, lithium salts, and phenothiazines and related drugs. For current *BNF* guidelines see www.bnf.org

Antidepressants

Tricyclic and realted antidepressants tricyclic and related antidepressants cause dry mouth, coma of varying degree, hypotension, hypothermia, hyperreflexia, extensor plantar responses, convulsions, respiratory failure, cardiac conduction defects, and arrhythmias. Dilated pupils and urinary retention also occur. Metabolic acidosis may complicate severe poisoning; delirium with confusion, agitation, and visual and auditory hallucinations are common during recovery.

Transfer to hospital is strongly advised in case of poisoning *tricyclic and related antidepressants* but symptomatic treatment and activated charcoal can be given before transfer. Supportive measures to ensure a clear airway and adequate ventilation during transfer are mandatory). Intravenous lorazepam or intravenous diazepam (preferably in emulsion form) may be required for control of convulsions. Although arrythmias are worrying, some will respond to correction of hypoxia and acidosis. The use of anti-arrhythmic drug is best avoided, but intravenous infusion of sodium bicarbonate can arrest arrhythmias or prevent them in those with an extended QRS duration. Diazepam given by mouth is usually adequate to sedate delirious patients but large doses may required.

Selective serotonin reuptake inhibitors (SSRIs)
Symptoms of poisoning by selective serotonin reuptake inhibitors include nausea, vomiting, agitation, tremor, nystagmus, drowsiness, and sinus tachycardia; convulsions may occur. Rarely, severe poisoning results in serotonin syndrome, with marked neuropsychiatric effects, neuromuscular hyperactivity, and autonomic instability; hyperthermia, rhabdomyolysis, renal failure, and coagulopathies may develop.

Management of SSRI poisoning is supportive. Activated charcoal given within 1 h of the overdose reduces absorbtion of the drug. Convulsions may be prevented with lorazepam or diazepam. Contact the National Poisons Information service for the management of hyperthermia or serotonin syndrome.

Lithium
Most cases of lithium intoxication occur as a complication of long-term therapy and are caused by reduced excretion of the drug due to a variety of factors including dehydration, deterioration of renal function, infections, and co-administration of diuretics or NSAIDs (or other drugs that interact). Acute deliberate overdoses may also occur with delayed onset of symptoms (12 hours or more) owing to slow entry of lithium into the tissues and continuing absorption from modified-release formulations.

The early clinical features are non-specific and may include apathy and restlessness which could be confused with mental changes arising from the patient's depressive illness. Vomiting, diarrhorea, ataxia, weakness, dysarthria, muscle twitching, and tremor may follow. Severe poisoning is asssociated with convulsions, coma, renal failure, electrolyte imbalance, dehydration, and hypotension.

Therapautic lithium concentrations are within the range of 0.4–1.0 mmol/litre; concerations in excess of 2.0 mmol/litre are usually associated with serious toxicity and such cases may need treatment with haemodialysis (if there is renal failure). In acute overdosage much higher serum concentrations may be present without features of toxicity and all that is usually necessary is to take measures to increase urine output (e.g. by increasing fluid intake but avoiding diuretics). Otherwise, treament is supportive with special regard to electrolyte balance, renal function, and controls of convulsions. Whole-bowl irrigation should be considered for significant ingestion, but advice should be sought from the National Poisons Information Service.

Phenothiazines and related drugs

Phenothiazines cause less depression of conciousness and respirations than other sedatives. Hypotension, hypothermia sinus tachycardia, and arrhythmias may complicate poisoning. Dystonic reactions can occur with therapeutic doses (particularly with prochlorperazine and trifluoperazine), and convulsions may occur in severe cases. Arrhythmias may respond to correction of hypoxia, acidosis, and other biochemical abnormalities, but specialist advice should be sought if arrhythmias form a prolonged QT interval; the use of some anti-arrhythmic drugs may worsen such arrhythmias. Dystonic reactions are abolished by injection of drugs such as benzatropine or diazepam.

Reference

1 Longmore M, Wilkinson I, Turmezei T, Cheung CK (2007). *Oxford Handbook of Clinical Medicine*, 7th edn. Oxford University Press: Oxford.

Resuscitation

Up to date recommendations for resuscitation have been provided in the European Resuscitation Council Guidelines for Resuscitation 2005[1]. For hospital inpatients, the algorithm shown in Fig. 2.3 should be used.

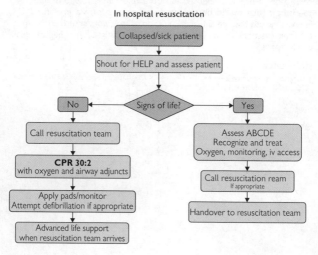

In hospital resuscitation

Collapsed/sick patient

Shout for HELP and assess patient

Signs of life?

No → Yes

No:
Call resuscitation team

CPR 30:2
with oxygen and airway adjuncts

Apply pads/monitor
Attempt defibrillation if appropriate

Advanced life support
when resuscitation team arrives

Yes:
Assess ABCDE
Recognize and treat
Oxygen, monitoring, iv access

Call resuscitation ream
If appropriate

Handover to resuscitation team

Fig. 2.3 Algorithm for resuscitation of hospital inpatients. Reproduced with kind permission from Nolan et al. (2005)[1]. Copyright European Resuscitation Council—www.erc.edu.

An advanced life support (ALS) cardiac arrest algorithm[1] is summarized in Fig. 2.4.

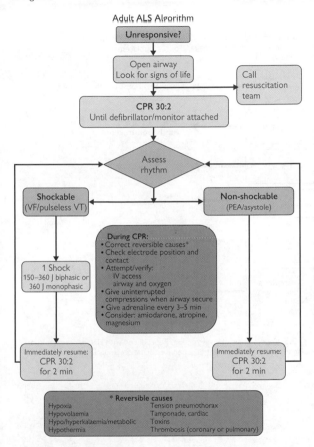

Fig. 2.4 Adult advanced cardiac arrest life support (ALS) algorithm. Reproduced with kind permission from Nolan *et al.* (2005)[1]. Copyright European Resuscitation Council—www.erc.edu.

Airway management and ventilation are key aspects of resuscitation. Causes of airway obstruction[1] are summarized in Fig. 2.5.

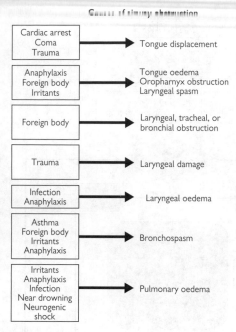

Fig. 2.5 Causes of airway obstruction. Reproduced with kind permission from Nolan et al.(2005)[1]. Copyright Europen Resuscitation Council—www.erc.edu.

After identifying any airway obstruction, basic airway management needs to be implemented immediately. The potentially life-saving procedures that should be used to increase airway patency are either tilting the head and lifting the chin, as shown in Fig. 2.6, or thrusting the jaw, shown in Fig. 2.7.

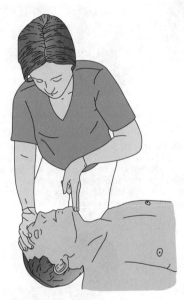

Fig. 2.6 Head tilt and chin lift. Reproduced with kind permission from Nolan et al. (2005)[1].

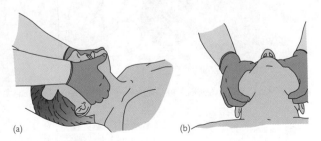

(a)   (b)

Fig. 2.7 Jaw thrust. Reproduced with kind permission from Nolan et al. (2005)[1].

An oropharyngeal airway may need to be inserted to keep the airway patent. This is shown in Fig. 2.8.

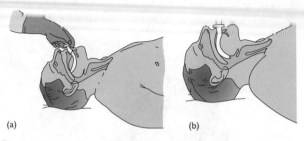

(a)   (b)

Fig. 2.8 Insertion of an oropharyngeal airway. Reproduced with kind permission from Nolan et al. (2005)[1].

Artificial ventilation may be provided using a mouth-to-mask technique, as shown in Fig. 2.9, in which both hands should be used to ensure the best possible seal with the face of the patient. A better technique is the use of a self-inflating bag by two people, as shown in Fig. 2.10, in which one person uses both hands to hold the mask over the face while applying jaw thrust, while the other person regularly squeezes the bag to provide ventilation.

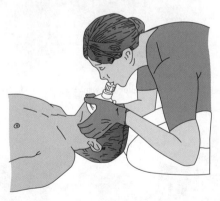

Fig. 2.9 Mouth-to-mask ventilation. Reproduced with kind permission from Nolan et al. (2005)[1].

A better, and more efficient, alternative is to use a laryngeal mask airway with a self-inflating bag. If this airway can be inserted without delay, then the current European Resuscitation Council Guidelines for Resuscitation recommend that it is preferable to avoid bag–mask ventilation altogether in favour of using the laryngeal mask airway plus self-inflating bag. Note that this method involves the use of an inflated cuff seal for the laryngeal opening, as shown in Fig. 2.11 and described by Nolan et al. (2005)[1].

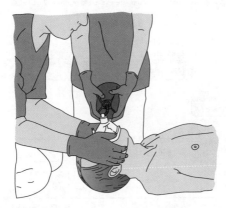

Fig. 2.10 Bag-mask ventilation by two people. Reproduced with kind permission from Nolan et al. (2005)[1].

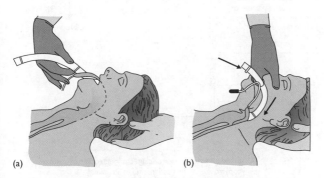

Fig. 2.11 Insertion of a laryngeal mask airway. Reproduced with kind permission from Nolan et al. (2005)[1].

When resuscitating a live patient with a heart rate noted to be less than 60 beats per min, the current European Resuscitation Council Guidelines for Resuscitation recommended procedures shown in the algorithm in Fig. 2.12 should be followed.

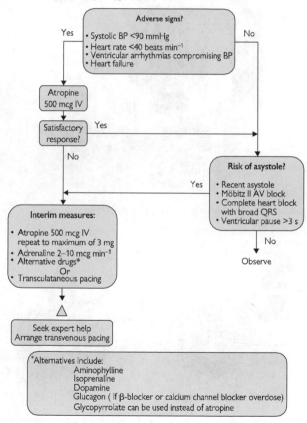

Bradycardia algorithm

(includes rates inappropriately slow for haemodynamic state)

If appropriate, give oxygen, cannulate a vein, and record a 12-lead ECG

Adverse signs?

Yes / No

- Systolic BP <90 mmHg
- Heart rate <40 beats min^{-1}
- Ventricular arrhythmias compromising BP
- Heart failure

Atropine
500 mcg IV

Satisfactory response? — Yes

No

Risk of asystole?

Yes

- Recent asystole
- Möbitz II AV block
- Complete heart block with broad QRS
- Ventricular pause >3 s

No

Observe

Interim measures:

- Atropine 500 mcg IV repeat to maximum of 3 mg
- Adrenaline 2–10 mcg min^{-1}
- Alternative drugs*

Or

- Transcutaneous pacing

Seek expert help
Arrange transvenous pacing

*Alternatives include:
Aminophylline
Isoprenaline
Dopamine
Glucagon (if β-blocker or calcium channel blocker overdose)
Glycopyrrolate can be used instead of atropine

Fig. 2.12 Algorithm for resuscitation in bradycardia. Reproduced with kind permission from Nolan et al. (2005).[1] Copyright European Resuscitation Council—www.erc.edu.

The corresponding European Resuscitation Council Guidelines for Resuscitation algorithm for tachycardia is given in Fig. 2.13.

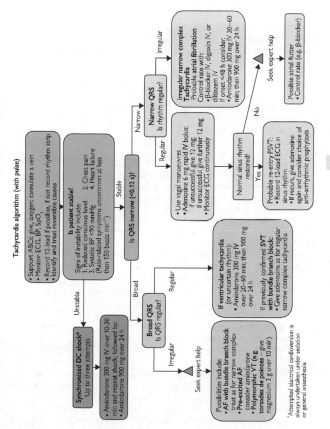

Fig. 2.13 Algorithm for resuscitation in tachycardia. Reproduced with kind permission from Nolan et al. (2005).[1] Copyright European Resuscitation Council—www.erc.edu.

Reference

1 Nolan JP, Deakin CD, Soar J, Böttiger BW, Smith G (2005). European Resuscitation Council Guidelines for Resuscitation 2005. Section 4. Adult advanced life support. *Resuscitation* **67**(Suppl. 1): S39–86.

☼ Wernicke's encephalopathy

This is most commonly seen in the context of drug- and alcohol-related disorders.

Clinical features

The most important clinical classical triad of Wernicke's encephalopathy, which is an acute neuropsychiatric disorder, are:

- Ophthalmoplegia—commonly affecting the external recti
- Nystagmus
- Ataxia
  Associated features which may also occur include:
- Clouding of consciousness
- Peripheral neuropathy
  Other ocular signs which may occur include:
- Ptosis
- Altered pupil reactions.

However, it is important to note that this syndrome may present without the full complement of classical features.

This is a psychiatric/medical emergency. Failure to diagnose Wernicke's encephalopathy and institute adequate parenteral treatment (see below) results in death in around one-fifth of patients, with three-quarters being left with permanent brain damage involving severe short-term memory loss (Korsakoff's psychosis)[1].

The Royal College of Physicians' Report on Alcohol[2] states the following in respect of potential sufferers of Wernicke's encephalopathy who turn up at accident and emergency (A&E) departments:

> Most alcohol-dependent patients presenting to A&E will spontaneously leave on sobering up. The common signs of [Wernicke's encephalopathy]—confusion, ataxia, and varying levels of impaired consciousness—are difficult or impossible to differentiate from drunkenness. The eye signs (ophthalmoplegia/nystagmus) are present in <30% of cases. Because of this, [Wernicke's encephalopathy] may go unrecognized if not considered, e.g. in the affluent or elderly.

> Heavy drinkers presenting to A&E—often collapsed and/or with a head injury—require repeated neurological assessment. The intoxicated patient who does not recover fully and spontaneously may be suffering from [Wernicke's encephalopathy]. Only if such a patient is admitted will full assessment be possible and further treatment be practical. There is no simple blood test to determine patients at risk of [Wernicke's encephalopathy].

Aetiology

The cause of Wernicke's encephalopathy is deficiency of thiamine (vitamin B_1). In turn, this can cause damage to those parts of the brain which are particularly thiamine-dependent. The mechanisms may include impairment of the following thiamine-dependent enzymes and systems[2]:

- Transketolase activity in the pentose phosphate pathway
- The maintenance of myelin sheaths in the nervous system
- Lipid metabolism
- Glucose metabolism
- Branched-chain amino acid biosynthesis
- Pyruvate conversion to acetyl CoA, leading to increased lactic acid synthesis
- α-Ketoglutarate conversion to succinate, with glutamate accumulation possibly increasing the production of free radicals.

In sum, the increased cellular metabolic demand leads to a cellular energy deficit, focal acidosis, regional increase in glutamate, and ultimately cell death[1,2].

The most common cause (around 90%) in the western world is alcohol abuse. (The term alcoholic encephalopathy has also been used in place of Wernicke's encephalopathy.). Other causes include[2,3]:

- Stomach lesions—such as gastric carcinoma, leading to malabsorption
- Duodenal lesions, leading to malabsorption
- Jejunal lesions, leading to malabsorption
- Hyperemesis
- Starvation
- Carbohydrate loading intravenously/orally when thiamine stores are minimal
- Chronic renal failure
- Hyperalimentation
- AIDS
- Drug misuse
- Genetic abnormality of transketolase enzyme.

Investigations

As mentioned above, there are no simple blood tests for diagnosing Wernicke's encephalopathy, which is essentially a clinical diagnosis. Non-routine blood investigation results which may be seen (and which in any case are not likely to be available in an emergency) are:

- A decrease in erythrocyte transketolase activity
- An increase in plasma pyruvate.

Management

Admission to an acute medical ward is indicated for giving thiamine replacement in adequate amounts parenterally to avoid irreversible brain damage (Korsakoff's psychosis); consider also magnesium, vitamin B6 and nicotinic acid deficiencies[2]. In the UK, the only parenteral high potency B-complex vitamin preparation which is licensed is Pabrinex®. Every 10 mL (two ampoules) of the intravenous version of this preparation contain:

- Vitamin B_1 (thiamine hydrochloride) 250 mg
- Vitamin C (ascorbic acid) 500 mg
- Anhydrous glucose 1 g
- Nicotinamide 160 mg
- Vitamin B_6 (pyridoxine hydrochloride) 50 mg
- Vitamin B_2 (riboflavin) 4 mg.

Always check the latest formulary guidelines (e.g. the *British National Formulary*) for the dosage guide. It is important to give intravenous doses as a slow infusion over at least 10 min. Also, as there is a risk of anaphylaxis occurring with parenteral B vitamins, they should be administered only in circumstances in which resuscitation facilities are readily available.

Oral niacin is poorly absorbed, and should only be used after an appropriate parenteral regimen has been completed.

References

1 Thomson AD, Marshall EJ (2006). The natural history and pathophysiology of Wernicke's encephalopathy and Korsakoff's psychosis. *Alcohol and Alcoholism* **41**: 151–8.
2 Thomson AD, Cook CCH, Touquet R, Henry JA (2002). The Royal College of Physicians report on alcohol: guidelines for managing Wernicke's encephalopathy in the accident and emergency department. *Alcohol and Alcoholism* **37**: 513–21.
3 Puri BK, Laking PJ, Treasaden IH (2002). *Textbook of Psychiatry*, 2nd edn. Churchill Livingstone: Edinburgh.

☠ Acute severe asthma

Asthma affects between 5 and 8% of the population. Acute severe asthma is a medical emergency which should ideally be treated in a medical hospital ward.

Presentation
Acute shortness of breath and wheeze. It is easy to underestimate its severity.

History
- Current treatment
- Previous episodes—their severity, need for inpatient treatment, best peak expiratory flow rate.

Investigations
- Peak expiratory flow rate
- Arterial blood gases
- Chest X-ray, including detection of infection or pneumothorax
- FBC
- U&Es.

Features of a severe attack
- Unable to talk properly
- High respiratory rate initially (>25 breaths per min), but may become feeble with cyanosis and lack of breath sounds and a silent chest
- Increased pulse rate but may develop bradycardia and/or hypotension
- Exhaustion, confusion, or coma
- Reduced peak expiratory flow rate (<50%).

Treatment
Treat immediately in severe asthma with high-dose oxygen, salbutamol (β_2-agonist) nebulizer, and steroids.

☠ Diabetic ketoacidosis and other diabetic emergencies

Diabetic ketoacidosis is a medical emergency which may occur not only in recognized diabetic patients, but also as a result of pharmacotherapy with atypical antipsychotics. The management may be particularly problematic in the following psychiatric groups:
- Old age psychiatry patients
- Chronic psychotic patients
- Juvenile diabetic patients in contact with a child and adolescent mental health service (CAMHS).

Although uncommon, the seriousness of diabetic ketoacidosis makes this such an important condition that one should, at least, be familiar with its treatment[1]. The ideal setting for the emergency treatment is a medical ward.

Features
- Only occurs in type 1 diabetes mellitus and may be its initial presentation
- Precipitants may include infection, surgery, myocardial infarction, and insufficient insulin dose, for example as a result of poor compliance with medication
- Polyuria, polydipsia, lethargy, anorexia, hyperventilation, characteristic ketotic breath, abdominal pain, dehydration, and vomiting
- In severe cases, coma may occur.

Management
- Establish IV access and rehydrate (dehydration is more life-threatening than hyperglycaemia)
- Blood tests, including glucose, FBC, U&Es, bicarbonate, blood gases, and blood culture
- Soluble insulin IV if plasma glucose >20 mM
- Test urine for ketones and infection
- Chest X-ray.

The following brief protocols describe the management of hypoglycaemic coma, hyperglycaemic hyperosmolar non-ketotic coma and hyperlactataemia.

Hypoglycaemic coma
There is often a rapid onset. Aggression and other disturbed behaviour may herald its onset. Tachycardia, sweating, and seizures may occur. Immediate treatment is either with IV dextrose or IV/IM glucagon. Give sugar-rich drinks and food upon regaining consciousness.

Hyperglycaemic hyperosmolar non-ketotic coma
This condition, which only occurs in type 2 diabetes mellitus, and particularly affects the elderly, is also known by the acronym HONK. Onset is gradual with marked dehydration and hyperglycaemia (>35 mM), without ketosis. There is a high risk of deep vein thrombosis, and so anticoagulation with heparin is required. Treatment otherwise is by rehydration and, later, insulin, if required.

Hyperlactataemia (blood lactate >5 mM)

Serious but rare complication of diabetes mellitus which may follow septicaemia or biguanide use. Administer oxygen, treat any infection, and refer to a specialist.

Reference

1 Nasrallah HA, Newcomer JW (2004). Atypical antipsychotics and metabolic dysregulation: evaluating the risk/benefit equation and improving the standard of care. *Journal of Clinical Psychopharmacology* **24**(Suppl. 1): S7–14.

☠ Notifiable diseases

As of January 2006, in the UK the following diseases were notifiable to Local Authority Proper Officers under the Public Health (Infectious Diseases) Regulations 1988:

- Acute encephalitis
- Acute poliomyelitis
- Anthrax
- Cholera
- Diphtheria
- Dysentery
- Food poisoning
- Leptospirosis
- Malaria
- Measles
- Meningitis—meningococcal, pneumococcal, *Haemophilus influenzae*, viral, other specified, unspecified
- Meningococcal septicaemia (without meningitis)
- Mumps
- Ophthalmia neonatorum
- Paratyphoid fever
- Plague
- Rabies
- Relapsing fever
- Rubella
- Scarlet fever
- Smallpox
- Tetanus
- Tuberculosis
- Typhoid fever
- Typhus fever
- Viral haemorrhagic fever
- Viral hepatitis—hepatitis A (HAV), hepatitis B (HBV), hepatitis C (HCV), other
- Whooping cough
- Yellow fever.

Leprosy is also notifiable, directly to the Health Protection Agency and its Centre for Infections and its IM&T department.

☠ Needlestick injuries

These may follow either professional accidents or deliberate harm by possibly infected individuals. The main risks are of infection with hepatitis B, hepatitis C, and HIV. The key management points are:

- Wear gloves if treating someone else's injury
- Clean wound with soap and water
- Ensure tetanus and hepatitis B cover
- Follow local guidelines if the patient is suspected of being HIV-positive. Prophylaxis is most effective if administered within an hour of exposure but may still be worthwhile up to a fortnight later. Use barrier contraception and do not donate blood until HIV seroconversion is ruled out
- A blood sample should be taken and stored for possible future baseline serology
- Refer to the local occupational health department if the incident took place in a hospital
- Offer follow-up counselling
- Be aware of local policies and procedures regarding needlestick injuries, as these may help prevent such incidents occurring.

☠ Human bite wounds

Occasionally a psychiatric patient may bite the attending doctor or another person such as another patient on a ward. There is a risk of bacterial infection of puncture wounds and/or contaminated crush injuries. Bacterial infection is particularly likely in those suffering from alcoholism or diabetes mellitus, or those who are otherwise immunocompromised.

If a fracture or joint involvement is suspected, then an X-ray may be indicated. An X-ray may also reveal the presence of one or more teeth belonging to the assailant.

The key management issues are:

- Debride and clean with normal saline
- Refer tendon or joint injuries to a specialist
- Do not attempt to close a puncture wound before adequate irrigation
- Ensure tetanus and hepatitis B cover
- Consider the risk of infection with hepatitis B, hepatitis C, and HIV, and manage accordingly (see 📖 Needlestick injuries p. 49)
- Refer to a specialist, who will advise on the appropriateness of further treatment, including antibiotics.

Psychiatric symptoms and syndromes presenting as emergencies

Acute psychoses 52
Endocrinopathies 56
Disorders presenting with anxiety and panic 58
Depressive and dysphoric symptomatology 62
Catatonic patients 64

☼ Acute psychoses

A psychosis is a severe mental illness with disorder of thinking and perception, with loss of contact with reality and of insight. This can present as 'odd', hostile, difficult-to-control behaviour. The patient is often very frightened by his/her unusual experiences, and this can limit engagement with professionals. Acute psychosis is a common psychiatric emergency that may present to any health service, not merely psychiatric services. Acute psychosis may commonly be compounded by comorbidity which increases with age, e.g. physical illness. Positive psychotic symptoms include delusions, unshakeable false beliefs out of keeping with the patient's background, and hallucinations, sensory perceptions experienced in the absence of a real stimulus, e.g. voices, visions.

Clinical features

Symptoms and signs of psychosis include[1]:
- Positive symptoms
  - Delusions
  - Hallucinations
  - Formal thought disorder
- Negative symptoms
  - Flat affect
  - Poverty of thought
  - Lack of motivation
  - Social withdrawal
- Cognitive symptoms
  - Distractibility
  - Impaired working memory
  - Impaired executive function
- Mood symptoms
  - Depression
  - Elevation (hypomania/mania)
- Anxiety/panic/perplexity
- Aggression/hostility/suicidal behaviour.

Aetiology

Primary functional psychotic disorders:
- Schizophrenia
- Bipolar disorder
  - Mania
  - Hypomania (elation without psychotic symptoms)
- Depression
- Schizophreniform disorder
- Schizoaffective (schizomood) disorder (combination at the same time of schizophreniform and mood symptomatology)
- Delusional disorder
- Acute and transient psychotic disorders.
Secondary (organic) psychotic disorders:
- Dementia
- Acute confusional state

- Psychosis resulting from an organic (physical) disorder
- Alcohol-induced
- Drug induced

Schizophrenia

A psychosis which usually develops a chronic course characterized by positive and negative psychotic symptoms. Characteristic first-rank Schneiderian positive psychotic symptoms of schizophrenia which should be present for at least a month include:

- Delusions of passivity (that others are controlling the patient's actions, body, and feelings)
- Delusions of thought interference, including of insertion, broadcast and withdrawal
- Thought echo (echo de la pensée), where a patient hears his or her own thoughts
- Third-person auditory hallucinations, in which voices speak about the patient and can include a running commentary.

In addition, thought disorder (illogical thinking) is a characteristic of schizophrenia.

Assessment/investigations

A detailed history, mental state examination, physical examination, and appropriate investigations, as outlined in Chapter 1, are required. Specific investigations include:

- *Blood tests and full blood count.* This could indicate anaemia, infection, with a raised white cell count or a low count in those taking clozapine; raised mean corpuscular volume (MCV) in longstanding alcohol misuse.
- *Urea and electrolytes* may indicate dehydration or renal impairment.
- *Random blood glucose.* If raised could indicate diabetes which may compound future prescription of antipsychotics. Required before the prescription of olanzapine.
- *Liver function tests.* Raised GGT in alcohol misuse. Intravenous drug users are often positive for hepatitis C antibodies.
- *Other blood tests*, e.g. thyroid function, HIV testing if indicated.
- *Urine drug screen.* Evidence suggests this should be undertaken even in cases where it appears very unlikely such an individual would have taken drugs. Detects illicit and also legal (benzodiazepine and alcohol) drugs.
- *Pregnancy test*, which may have implications for future management.
- An *ECG* helps exclude ischaemic and other heart diseases. Caution is required in the use of antipsychotic drugs in those with cardiac disease, including because of prolongation of QTc interval.
- *EEG.* Temporal lobe epilepsy may in particular present with auditory and visual hallucinations, but epilepsy may be associated with psychosis.
- *Brain imaging.* CT or, if available, MRI, which shows more subtle changes, is definitely indicated where there are neurological symptoms or atypical presentations, but many consider such an investigation is prudent in all first episodes of psychosis.

Management

As an individual with acute psychosis can be impulsive, unpredictable, and a risk to themselves and/or others, care should be taken to see such individuals in designated safe and secure interview rooms with alarm systems in hospital or mental health facilities. Patients should ideally never be seen alone in their homes. Such measures are especially important when seeing new referrals previously unseen. Information from relatives, staff and, where relevant, ward observation sheets, can be invaluable in 'getting the whole picture'. If an organic cause is found for the psychosis, then this should be treated.

Patients with a first episode of acute psychosis are considered best treated by the new specialist multidisciplinary early intervention teams that deliver a psychosocial intervention as well as standard drug treatments. Such services are even considered appropriate where the first episode of psychosis is induced by a substance misuse. It has been argued that low dose well tolerated atypical oral antipsychotic medication at the time of the first episode will increase medium-term compliance, which in turn improves the prognosis by reducing the risk of future relapses. Overall complete remission without relapse of acute psychosis is seen in about a quarter of patients.

An organic cause, if found, should be treated.

It is good to try to explain, in simple terms, the disorder and your management decisions regarding admission/community treatment and specific pharmacological treatments to the patient, even if they do not appear to be able to understand everything that you say. Reassure the patient that you understand that their current condition might be scaring them, but that they are likely to become better with the treatment you are instigating. Even if not consciously acknowledged, your explanations and reassurance may be helpful for the patient at an unconscious level.

Inpatient admission, if necessary using the mental health legislation (see Chapter 20), may be required for patients who are:
- Hostile/aggressive—and perhaps even homicidal
- Suicidal
- Sexually disinhibited
- Intent on committing a dangerous act such as fire-setting.

The management recommendations of Keks and Blashki[1] are reproduced in Table 3.1. Note that if rapid tranquillization is required, then parenteral lorazepam may be a better choice than diazepam, which is slower in onset and has a longer duration of action. Local policies/Trust guidelines should be referred to as they may be helpful .

Table 3.1 Managing acute psychoses. Reprduced with permission from *Australian Family Physician*

Assess danger to self/others and need for hospitalization

Assess physical state and consider possibility of substance abuse

Consider specialist treatment options (e.g. psychiatrist, involvement of mobile community outreach psychiatric services)

Antipsychotic medication:

- Risperidone 1 mg twice per day, increasing over a few days to 2 mg twice per day
- Olanzapine 5–10 mg at night
- Quetiapine 25 mg twice per day (day 1), 50 mg twice per day (day 2), 100 mg twice per day (day 3), 100 mg morning and 200 mg at night (day 4), 200 mg twice per day (day 5)
- Amisulpride 300–400 mg twice per day
- Aripiprazole 15 mg per day

If response is inadequate in 3 weeks, the dose can be increased (unless significant extrapyramidal side-effects occur) to:

- Risperidone to 2 mg twice per day, up to 3 mg twice per day
- Olanzapine to 20 mg at night
- Quetiapine 400–750 mg per day
- Amisulpride 400–800 mg twice per day
- Aripiprazole 20–30 mg per day

Treat anxiety, agitation, and insomnia with short-term diazepam, repeated as required. Quetiapine and chlorpromazine can also be used

A manic presentation may require addition of a mood stabilizer (e.g. lithium, valproate, carbamazepine)

If depression persists, adjunctive antidepressants may be necessary

Consider the use of long-acting injectable risperidone if adherence is unlikely despite psychosocial interventions, or the patient fails to achieve optimal response from oral therapy

Engage the patient in supportive psychotherapy and case management. Family therapy and cognitive behaviour therapy may be indicated

Consider social interventions: housing options, resources, social supports

Evaluate functional status and consider vocational rehabilitation options

Reference

1 Keks N, Blashki G (2006). The acutely psychotic patient: assessment and initial management. *Australian Family Physician* **35**: 90–4.

☠ Endocrinopathies

☠ Myxoedema coma

Hypothyroidism may present with symptomatology similar to that seen in depression, (hypo)mania, and schizophrenia (myxoedema madness). Following infection, myocardial infarction, a cerebrovascular accident, or trauma, a hypothyroid patient may enter into a myxoedema coma. This is a medical emergency, in which the patient may suffer from:

- Hypothermia
- Hyporeflexia
- Bradycardia
- Seizures
- Coma.

Patients should be urgently transferred to an intensive care unit for medical treatment.

☠ Thyrotoxic storm

Hyperthyroidism may present in adults with symptomatology similar to that seen in mood disorders, panic disorder, and generalized anxiety disorder. Following infection, myocardial infarction, trauma, or surgical or radioiodine treatment to reduce the hyperthyroidism, a patient may enter into a thyrotoxic storm (or hyperthyroid crisis). This is a medical emergency, in which the patient may suffer from:

- Pyrexia
- Mental confusion
- Agitation
- Tachycardia
- Atrial fibrillation
- An acute abdominal-like clinical picture
- Coma.

Urgent referral for medical treatment is required.

☠ Addisonian crisis

In Addison's disease (primary hypoadrenalism), the patient may suffer from similar symptoms to those that occur in depression. Such patients may be mistakenly diagnosed as suffering from depression for many years. Following infection, trauma or surgery, a patient with previously unrecognized Addison's disease may suffer from an Addisonian crisis with a presentation of either shock or hypoglycaemia. (Shock may manifest as tachycardia, mental confusion, weakness, postural hypotension, peripheral vasoconstriction, oliguria, and coma.) This is a medical emergency requiring urgent medical referral.

ⓘ Disorders presenting with anxiety and panic

Clinical features

Psychic symptoms of anxiety may be accompanied by somatic (bodily) symptoms. The well known somatic symptoms of anxiety include:

- Tremor
- Paraesthesia
- Choking
- Palpitations
- Chest pain
- Dry mouth
- Nausea
- Abdominal pain—'butterflies'
- Loose bowel motions
- Increased frequency of micturition.

Panic attacks are unexpected severe acute exacerbations of psychic and somatic anxiety symptoms with intense fear and dread. They are not triggered by situations, as is the case in phobias, and an individual cannot 'sit out' such an attack.

Aetiology

There are numerous organic conditions that present with anxiety. In these, anxiety may resolve with treatment of the primary problem. Some causes of anxiety are given in Table 3.2.

There are also many psychiatric causes of anxiety symptoms[1]. Primary diagnoses include:

- Generalized anxiety disorder
- Panic disorder
- Phobic disorders
- Obsessive-compulsive disorder
- Acute stress disorder
- Post-traumatic stress disorder.

These are often abnormal psychogenic reactions to stress in vulnerable personalities. Contact with reality and insight is maintained. These disorders relate to the general public's view of an individual suffering from 'nerves'.

Other diagnoses that can present with associated anxiety features include:

- Depressive disorder
- Schizophrenia
- Other paranoid psychoses
- Early dementia—e.g. catastrophic reactions upon psychometric testing
- Adjustment disorders.

Miscellaneous conditions presenting with anxiety include:

- Unexpressed complaints of physical illness, e.g. after discovering a breast lump
- Personal crisis
- Being bullied
- After encountering a major disaster.

Table 3.2 Causes of organic anxiety disorder. Reproduced from Puri BK et al. (2002). *Textbook of Psychiatry*, 2nd edn, with permission from Elsevier.

Psychoactive substance use	Alcohol and drug withdrawl Amphetamine and related sympathomimetics Cannabis
Intoxication	Drugs—penicillin, sulphonamides Caffeine and caffeine withdrawl Poisons—arsenic, mercury, organophosphates, phosphorus, benzene Aspirin intolerance
Intracranial causes	Brain tumours Head injury Migraine Cerebrovascular disease Subarachnoid haemorrhage Infections—encephalitis, neurosyphilis Multiple sclerosis Hepatolenticular degeneration (Wilson's disease) Huntington's disease Epilepsy
Endocrine	Pituitary dysfunction Thyroid dysfunction Parathyroid dysfunction Adrenal dysfunction Phaeochromocytoma Hypoglycaemia Virilzation disorders of females
Inflammatory disorders	Systemic lupus erythematosus Rheumatiod arthritis Polyarteritis nodosa Temporal arteritis
Vitamin deficiency	Vitamin B_{12} deficiency Pellagra (nicotinic acid deficiency)
Other systemic disorders	Hypoxia Cardiovascular disease Cardiac arrhythmias Pulmonary insufficiency Anaemia Carcinoid syndrome Systemic neoplasia Febrile illnesses and chronic infections Porphyria Infectious mononucleosis (glandular fever) Posthepatic syndrome Uraemia Premenstrual syndrome

Hyperventilation (either tachypnoea or hyperpnoea) may result in a respiratory alkalosis and hypocalcaemia. Anxiety is the commonest cause. Symptoms specifically caused by hyperventilation include:

- Palpitations
- Dizziness
- Faintness
- Tinnitus
- Chest pains
- Perioral paraesthesia
- Peripheral paraesthesia.

Assessment/investigations

A detailed history, mental state examination, physical examination, and appropriate investigations are required (see Chapter 1). Of the organic causes, it is particularly important to exclude hyperthyroidism, phaeochromocytoma, and hypoglycaemia.

Management

The management should, of course, be aimed at treating the underlying cause. In the short term, when asked to manage acute anxiety symptoms, the relevant elements of the following protocol can be followed:

- Explain the nature of the symptoms to the patient. They may be worried about somatic symptoms such as palpitations and chest pain, which may make some people feel that they are about to suffer from a heart attack, for example. An explanation of the effects of hyperventilation can be beneficial.
- Reassure the patient.
- Breathing exercises can be given. The patient should be encouraged not to hyperventilate, if necessary by making use of a paper bag into which the patient can re-breathe to help reduce the respiratory alkalosis that can worsen the condition.
- Relaxation techniques—these may involve progressive muscular relaxation.
- Positive reinforcing self-statements, which the patient can write down if they are unable to articulate them, for example owing to hyperventilation.

In the longer term, after the acute crisis is over, the patient may benefit from being referred for more formal psychological treatments.

Benzodiazepines are still the first choice when a rapid anxiolytic effect is required. They should be used judiciously in the lowest possible dose and only as required, rather than routinely. In the absence of anxiety they may merely result in sedation and increase the risk of dependency. They should not be prescribed as a hypnotic for more than 10 days or as an anxiolytic for more than 4 weeks. Prescribing for a period of even 2 weeks can be associated, on cessation, not only with the re-emergence of original symptoms, which the patient may blame on the drug, but also with rebound anxiety and insomnia. Patients should therefore be warned that they may find it difficult to sleep for a few days after stopping benzodiazepine medication. Around one-third of long-term benzodiazepine users will experience withdrawal syndrome upon stopping benzodiazepines. The emergence of new neurotic symptoms, or any symptoms not part of the psychiatric disorder for which the benzodiazepine was prescribed, e.g. neurological symptoms or lippry hallucinations, are indicative of dependency.

It is therefore important to review all short-term benzodiazepine prescriptions, advise the patient of this, document this clearly and let the patient know that this has been done specifically.

Reference

1 Puri BK, Laking PJ, Treasaden IH (2002). *Textbook of Psychiatry*, 2nd edn. Churchill Livingstone: Edinburgh.

① Depressive and dysphoric symptomatology

Depression can present with varying degrees of severity and a decision to manage the patient in an inpatient setting may be guided by whether the patient can safely sustain themselves in the community without serious risk to their health, safety, or to others.

Admission to a psychiatric ward, if necessary compulsorily using mental health legislation, may be required in cases of patients with depressive symptomatology who are:

• Actively suicidal/at risk
• Not taking care of themselves—for example, not eating (look for weight loss), not drinking sufficient amounts of fluid (look for dehydration), being unkempt, being at risk from an infection owing to poor personal and/or residential hygiene
• Homicidal—for example, suicidal patients can enter into pacts, elderly depressed people might wish to kill their spouse/partner first, while depressed mothers might wish to kill their children before committing suicide
• Suffering from delusions and/or hallucinations
• Homeless and/or otherwise without an adequate network of social support.

Aetiology

In addition to important psychiatric diagnoses such as mood disorder and schizophrenia, it is always important to bear in mind that there are many organic causes of mood disorder (depression or (hypo)mania), such as those given in Table 3.3.

Assessment/investigations

A detailed history, mental state examination, physical examination, and appropriate investigations are required (see Chapter 1).

Management

The decision as to whether or not to admit the patient to a psychiatric ward can be made partly on the basis of the criteria given above. There may be other cases in which admission is also advisable, such as cases of depressive symptomatology in which the next of kin or other carer(s) are unable to look after the patient at home any more. Inpatient admission may allow the patient to feel a sense of relief at having their illness contained in some way. More often, however, patients continue to be suicidal. In such cases, regular close observations of the patients need to be requested of the psychiatric nursing staff, and patients should be denied access to all potential means of suicide, such as belts, shoelaces, telephone cords, wires, pyjama cords, and loose sheeting (by means of which a patient could be hanged), and knives, electrical sockets, and wiring.

Elderly patients are at risk of hypothermia/dehydration owing to possible self-neglect.

Table 3.3 Causes of organic mood disorders. Reproduced from Puri BK et al. (2002). *Textbook of Psychiatry*, 2nd edn, with permission from Elsevier.

Psychoactive substance use	Amphetamine and related sympathomimetics Hallucinogens, e.g. LSD
Medication	Corticosteroids Levodopa Centrally acting antihypertensives—clonidine, methyldopa, reserpine and rauwolfia alkaloids Cycloserine Osetrogens—hormone replacement theraphy, oral contraceptives Clomifene
Endrocrine disorders	Hypothyroidism, hyperthyroidism Addison's disease Cushing's syndrome Hypoglycemia, diabetes mellitus Hypeparathyroidism Hypopituitarism
Other systematic disorders	Pernicious anaemia Hepatic failure Renal failure Rheumatoid arthritis Systemic lupus erythematosus Neoplasia—particularly carcinoma of the pancreas, carcinoid syndrome Viral infections—e.g. influenza, pneumonia, infectious mononucleosis (glandular fever), hepatitis
Intracranial causes	Brain tumours Head injury Parkison's disease Infections, e.g. neurosyphilis

Antidepressant medication may need to be (re-)started. In urgent cases, electroconvulsive therapy or repetitive transcranial magnetic stimulation may need to be considered; the latter is very safe, but currently tends only to be available in research centres.

The long-term management will require a plan that takes into account the relevant risk factors already identified. Always bear in mind the possible need for social assistance (e.g. with housing, income support, day care, home help) and the need to liaise with social services, the patient's general practitioner, occupational therapy, and the patient's psychiatric team (if it is not yours).

:◉: Catatonic patients

Clinical features

Catatonia was described by Karl Kahlbaum[1] as a cyclic, alternating, linear disease with consecutive stages of depression, mania, stupor, confusion, plus or minus dementia. In addition, several movement abnormalities were identified. These days, the following signs are recognized as occurring in catatonia[2]:

- Immobility/stupor—extreme passivity, marked hypokinesia
- Mutism—including inaudible whispering
- Negativism—a motiveless resistance to commands and attempts to be moved
- Oppositionism/gegenhalten—resistance to passive movement which increases with the force exerted
- Posturing—the person adopts an inappropriate or bizarre bodily posture continuously for a long period
- Catalepsy and waxy flexibility (*cerea flexibilitas*)—there is a feeling of plastic resistance resembling the bending of a soft wax rod as the examiner moves part of the person's body; that body part then remains 'moulded' in the new position
- Automatic obedience—exaggerated cooperation with instructed movements
- Echopraxia—automatic imitation by the person of another person's movements; it occurs even when the person is asked not to do so
- Echolalia—automatic imitation by the person of another person's speech; it occurs even when the person is asked not to do so
- Muscle rigidity—increasing muscle tone giving rise to rigid posturing
- Verbigeration—continuous and directionless repetition of single words or phrases
- Withdrawal/refusal to eat or drink—turning away from the examiner, making no eye contact, refusing to take food or drink when these are offered.

Aetiology

The most important causes of catatonic features as seen in psychiatric practice include:
- Psychiatric (functional)
  - Schizophrenia
  - Mood disorders
  - Antipsychotic drugs
- Organic
  - Encephalitis
  - Carbon monoxide poisoning
  - Serum potassium imbalance (periodic paralysis).

Assessment/investigations/management

The following management procedure is mainly based on that suggested by Pommepuy and Januel[2]:

- Withhold neuroleptic (antipsychotic) medication, since these drugs can be dangerous to take when catatonic symptoms and signs have developed.
- Carry out a full physical examination and investigations to exclude treatable physical disorders—these should include standard laboratory blood tests, urinary drug screening, electroencephalography, and cerebral imaging (computerized tomography or magnetic resonance imaging).
- A trial of lorazepam. Pommepuy and Januel[2] recommend this as a safe intervention which is effective in around 80% of patients. They recommend an initial oral challenge of 2.5 mg lorazepam and rate catatonic signs after the first hour. If necessary, they recommend a daily dose of 3 mg lorazepam for up to 6 days, followed by a progressive reduction in daily dose.
- If the patient fails to respond to lorazepam, then electroconvulsive therapy is recommended.

If the patient has malignant catatonia, in which there is autonomic instability, with labile blood pressure and hyperthermia, then urgent electroconvulsive therapy is required. The mortality rate from malignant catatonia[2] may be around 25%.

References

1 Kahlbaum KL (1874). (Translation by Levi Y, Pridon T 1973) *Catatonia*. Johns Hopkins University Press: Baltimore.
2 Pommepuy N, Januel D (2002). Catatonia: resurgence of a concept. A review of the international literature. *Encephale* **28**: 481–92.

Chapter 4

Aggression and violence

Schizophrenia and violence 70
Warning signs 70
Terminology 70
Checklist to aid assessment and management 71
Risk of violence among psychiatric inpatients 72
Assessment 74
Risk factors for violence have been recently
    usefully summarized 75
Management 77
Summary of management of aggression and violence 82
Safety in outpatient settings 84
Safety in the community 85
Burns 86

Aggression is a bio/psycho/social/environmental phenomenon. Biochemical abnormalities cause psychological symptoms, but also psychological events, e.g. severe abuse in childhood may cause neurobiological, including biochemical, abnormalities in adults. There may be a normal inborn assertiveness and indeed normal aggression as shown in all members of society. Pathological aggression is excessive in degree and secondary to background and upbringing, with or without mental disorder (Table 4.1 and 4.2).

Table 4.1 Violence and psychiatric disorder

Non-psychiatric causes—social
Economic
Criminal e.g. drug dealing
Cultural e.g. subcultures

Psychiatric causes
Violence or threats of viloence in 40% pre-admission
Schizophrenia —paranoid and non-paranoid
Maina, hypomania but also depression
Alcohol abuse and withdrawal
Drug abuse and withdrawal
Hallucinogens, PCP
Benzodiazepine withdrawal
Organic mental disorder and brain damage, epilepsy, especially TLE, dementia
Personality disorder, particularly antisocial, impulsive, and borderline
Learning disability
Child and adolescent behaviour disorders
Post—traumatic stress disorder
Dissociative states

Intra-familial
Spousal abuse
Child abuse
Elder abuse

Table 4.2 Models and factors in violence

Biological	Fight or flight response
	Males and young more violent
	Testosterone levels
	Reduced serotonin (5HT) levels in brain
Alcohol and drugs	50% violence follows alcohol abuse in UK
	Disinhibits
Psychological models	
1. Instrumental aggression	Learn to achieve ends by violence
2. Cognitive model	Look at world aggressively
3. Behavioural model	Inconsistent, erratic parental punishment
4. Social learning	Peer pressure/modelling (Bandura)
5. Status	Status of being violent
Psychodynamic models	
1. Freudian	Primary drive due to frustration
	Later, primary drive libido, aggression secondary drive
2. Kleinian	Annihilation anxiety
3. Kohut	Secondary to developmental insults or deprivations
4. Object relation school (Winnicott)	Aggression is creative another
5. Attachment theory	Insecurely attached infant, e.g. deprived or abused relates to others with hostility
Famliy factors	Physical abuse as child
	Parental discord and viloence
	Parental irritability, usually due to depression
Social models	Criminal, e.g. drug dealing
	Subcultural norm e.g. hells angels
	Pub brawls
	Sporting, political, and industrial violence
	Relative poverty and inequility
	Comparative anthropolgy e.g. Mead's studies
Environmental factors	Avoidence of frustration by well structured and staffed milieu and non-provocative regime
Psychiatric disorders	Schizophrenia, especially paranoid type
	Hypomania and mania more than depression
	Organic mental disorder
	Personality disorder
	Post-traumatic stress disorder

☼ Schizophrenia and violence

Research there is a consistent association between delusions and violence, particularly the following threat/control override symptoms which double the risk of violence[1]:

- Persecutory delusions
- Passivity delusions
- Thought insertion.

However, other risk factors for all, not just psychotic, patients may be relevant:

- Young
- Male
- Expressed threats
- Substance abuse
- History of personal deprivation and/or abuse.

Reference

1 Link BG, Stueve A (1994). Psychotic symptoms and violent/illegal behaviour of mental patients compared to community controls. In: Monahan J, Steadman HJ (eds). *Violence in Mental Disorder: Developments in Risk Assessment*. University of Chicago Press: Chicago, pp. 137–60.

☼ Warning signs

The Royal College of Psychiatrists (1996), in their paper *Assessment and Clinical Management of Risk of Harm to Other People*, have identified the following research-based warning signs of risk of violence:

- Beliefs of persecution, control by external forces
- Previous violence or suicide attempts
- Social restlessness
- Poor compliance with medication or treatment
- Substance abuse
- Hostility, suspiciousness, anger
- Threats.

Terminology

- *Aggression* refers to threats or acts of violence.
- *Violence* is action.
- *Dangerousness* is potential violence and is a matter of opinion.
- *Risk* is an elusive concept but ideally is a matter of statistical fact, a calculation of the probability of the potential occurrence of an adverse effect. It is now used in preference to dangerousness, as an individual is rarely dangerous all the time, but only in certain situations of increased risk.
- *Risk assessment* = practical risk assessment (history × mental state × environment) plus standard actuarial and dynamic risk assessment instruments, e.g. HCR-20. Risk assessment is incomplete without an appropriate risk management strategy.
- *Risk management* does not, however, equate with *risk elimination*.

Checklist to aid assessment and management

- Patient
  - Personality
  - Life experience
  - Recent severe stress
  - Substance abuse
  - Previous violence
  - Illness
    —poor compliance
    —recent cessation of treatment.
- Potential victims
  - Family
  - Intimates
  - Workmates
  - People in authority
  - Hospital/institution staff
  - Sex and age
- Environment
  - Interview room
  - Forgotten corridor
  - Lone assessor on dark housing estate
  - Loss of/poor accommodation
  - Weapons
  - Alcohol/drugs.

Psychiatric patients peak for violence at a later age than the general population.

'The best predictor of future behaviour is past behaviour' (after Kvaraceus 1954)[1].

However, this is:

- Based on non-psychiatric population
- Accounts for only 5% variance[2]
- History of previous violence required for inclusion in study
- Among psychotic, delusions of threat/control override better predictor (Hallucinations play a minimal role alone; although on occasions command hallucinations may be relevant).

Violence can occur in psychiatric ward settings or in general medical settings (especially critical care and elderly wards), the latter having less access to resources to deal with it.

References

1 Kvaraceus WC (1954). *The Community and the Delinquent.* World Book: Yonkers-on-Hudson.
2 Steadman HJ, Mulvey EP, Monahan J, Robbins PC, Appelbaum PS, Grisso T, *et al.* (1998). Violence by people discharged from acute psychiatric in-patient facilities and others in the same neighbourhoods. *Archives of General Psychiatry* **55**: 393–401.

① Risk of violence among psychiatric inpatients

For those recently admitted, about a half have thoughts of self-harm and a third have thoughts of violence to others. Rates are higher in the case of detained patients.

Imminent risk
- Intention (premeditation) to act on violent thoughts
- Threats to identifiable victims
- Access to potential victims
- Availability of or carrying weapons.

Always enquire into *circumstances of previous violence*, including previous convictions for violence.

Key risk factors
- Male if in community, but not among inpatients
- Young
- Lower socioeconomic class
- History of previous violence, including previous convictions for violence
- Substance misuse
- For mentally ill, acute positive psychotic symptoms, especially threat/control override delusions (e.g. paranoid delusions, delusions of passivity), are best predictors
- Violence or an offence = offender x victim x situation/environment.

NB. Offending is not a characteristic or diagnostic symptom of any mental illness.

Staff attitudes associated with violence
- Expectations of violence
- Rigid intolerance
- Authoritarian style.

Most assaults by a patient are provoked by interaction with staff.

However, conflicts arise over:
- Denial of privileges
- Denial of discharge
- Patient
  - Wants something that is not possible
  - Refuses to participate in required activities
  - Demands instant gratification
  - Demands instant emotional attention.

Preventable causes in psychiatric wards
The Royal College of Psychiatrists' Research Unit (2005)[1] has identified the following preventable causes of aggression and violence towards psychiatrists in psychiatric wards (see also Royal College of Psychiatrists, 2006[2]):
- Flaws in the design of inpatient units
- Inadequate staffing

- Over-reliance on agency staff
- Poor leadership
- Changes in the clinical mix —with a higher proportion of patients with dual diagnoses
- Overcrowding
- A higher prevalence of substance misuse
- High levels of boredom
- Dissatisfaction among staff with the appropriateness of training in the management of violence.

References

1 Royal College of Psychiatrists' Research Unit (2005). *The National Audit of Violence (2003–2005). Final Report.* Royal College of Psychiatrists: London.
2 Royal College of Psychiatrists (2006). *Safety for Psychiatrists.* Council Report CR134. Royal College of Psychiatrists: London.

Assessment

Diagnostic assessment

Rocca et al. (2006)[1] divide violence into:
- Cognitive violence
- Emotional violence.

Cognitive violence is usually more related to criminal attitude than to psychiatric disorders, while the opposite is true for emotional violence.[1,2] Rocca et al. (2006) suggest that the first step for the clinician should be to distinguish between these two types of violence; a medical/psychiatric diagnostic workup is particularly important, in order to select the most appropriate interventions. If possible, the vital signs should be checked, and a physical examination (or at least a visual examination) carried out. Toxicological screening and other blood investigations should also be carried out as soon as possible. A pregnancy test is appropriate for female patients in the reproductive age group.

The following diagnoses should be considered particularly[1]:
- Substance misuse disorders, including delirium—drug intoxication should be distinguished from drug withdrawal, so that an appropriate intervention is carried out
- General medical conditions, including delirium, dementia, and neuro-logical syndromes such as complex partial seizures, temporal lesions, frontal lesions and limbic lesions
- Psychiatric causes, which may or may not be comorbid with substance misuse or a general medical disorder. Particular disorders to consider include
  - First episode psychosis
  - Chronic schizophrenia with exacerbation
  - Mood disorders
  - Cluster B personality disorders
  - Panic disorder
  - Other acute anxiety disorders—including post-traumatic stress disorder.

Violence risk assessment

Factors associated with a risk of violence in psychiatric patients are given in Table 4.3.

Overall, the aim of a risk assessment is to answer how serious is the risk; that is:
- Its nature and magnitude
- Is it specific or general?
- Is it conditional or unconditional?
- Immediate, long term or volatile.

Have the individuals or situational risk factors changed: who might be at risk?

Table 4.3 Violence risk assessment[1]. Reproduced with permission from Elsevier

Risk of violence among psychiatric patients has been associated with the following factors

- Demographic—male, young (15–24 years old), poor, uneducated, unemployed, minority, no supportive social network

- Past history—early victimization, past violence, substance abuse, early onset, poor parental model

- Diagnostic—organic brain syndrome (including intoxications), personality disorder, psychosis, comorbidity with substance abuse

- Clinical features—command auditory hallucinations, paranoid delusions and suspiciousness, poor impulse control, poor insight and low adherence to treatment, low IQ score, low GAF score

- Psychological—low tolerence for frustration, criticism and interpersonal closeness, low self-esteem, tendency toward projection and externalization, anger, irritability, patient's previous methods of coping with similar stressors, motivation, and capacity to participate in the treament process.

References

1 Rocca P, Villari V, Bogetto F (2006). Managing the aggressive and violent patient in the psychiatric emergency. *Progress in Neuro-Psychopharmacology and Biological Psychiatry* **30**: 586–98.
2 Petit JR (2004). *Handbook of Emergency Psychiatry*. Lippincott, Williams and Wilkins: Philadelphia.

Risk factors for violence have been recently usefully summarized[1]

Demographic factors
- Male
- Young age
- Socially disadvantaged neighbourhoods
- Lack of social support
- Employment problems
- Criminal peer group.

Background history
- Childhood maltreatment
- History of violence
- First violent at young age
- History of childhood conduct disorder
- History of non-violent criminality.

Clinical history
- Psychopathy
- Substance abuse
- Personality disorder
- Schizophrenia
- Executive dysfunction
- Non-compliance with treatment.

Psychological and psychosocial factors

- Anger
- Impulsivity
- Suspiciousness
- Morbid jealousy
- Criminal/violent attitudes
- Command hallucinations
- Lack of insight.

Current 'context'

- Threats of violence
- Interpersonal discord/instability
- Availability of weapons.

Reference

1 National Mental Health Risk Management Programme (2007). *Best Practice in Managing Risk*. D.O.H.: London, Appendix 2.

ⓘ Management

Following a risk assessment (see above) a risk management plan should be developed to modify the risk factors and specify response triggers. This should ideally be agreed with the individual. Is there a need for:
- More frequent follow-up appointments
- An urgent care programme approach meeting
- Admission to hospital
- Detention under the Mental Health Act
- Physical security
- Observation and/or medication?

If the optimum plan cannot be undertaken, reasons for this should be documented and a back-up plan specified.

Risk assessments and risk management plans should be communicated to others on a 'need to know' basis. On occasions, patient confidentiality will need to be breached if there is immediate grave danger to others. The police can often do little unless there has been a specific threat to an individual, whereupon they may warn or charge the subject. Very careful consideration needs to be given before informing potential victims to avoid their unnecessary anxiety. Their safety is often best ensured by management of those who present the risk.

Management strategies for violence include:
- Priority: safety of the patient, other patients on the ward, staff
- Least restrictive methods
- Plan setting of management. If in a medical ward, may need either supervision on site by qualified mental health nursing staff or transfer to a psychiatric unit
- Protect yourself
- Alert police/security as appropriate in case of increased risk, e.g. if unsure of the presence of weapons.

Behavioural and environmental interventions are given in Table 4.4[1]; verbal approaches which should be used are given in Table 4.5[1], and variables relating to the patient–therapist relationship are summarized in Table 4.6[1].

Table 4.4 Behavioural and environmental interventions, Reproduced with permission from Elsevier

- Use a room or an area which is large and calm, and which is not isolated to allow others to come quickly if help is needed.

- You and the patient should be in such a position as to allow the both of you to reach the door easily; this must be open

- Choose as calm as possible an environment without intense stimulations or triggers

- The environment must be safe, without objects that can be potentially dangerous

- If a suitable room is not available use an open space

- keep your distance; do not get too close: the violent patient needs more room than others. Never approach the patient from behind or in a rough manner

- Never turn your back on the patient

- Do not be confrontational, do not look the in the eyes, try to assume a neutral facial expression and voice tone, and a relaxed body posture; avoid positions such as crossed arms or hands behind the back

- The patient does not have to be left alone

- If others represent a trigger for the patient's violence, ask them to leave the area

- Give information and support to raletives and significant others

- Perform a debriefing with the staff and, if possible, also with the patient

Table 4.5 Verbal approach. Reproduced with permission from Elsevier

- Introduce youself and explain what are you going to do

- Use easy words, short and clear sentences, and a calm manner

- Use a confidential but formal tone. Pay attention to be tuned

- Help the patient to understand what is happening and reassure him about the diagnostic and the therapeutic procedure he will undergo

- Help the patient to restore his orientation

- Prefer, at least at the beginning, alliance ori-ented questions and wait for more delicate issues

- When possible try to talk about the real moti-vations of the violence

- Set limits of acceptable behaviour and tell the patient that violations will not be allowed

- Encourage the verbal expression of feelings, states of mind, fantasies, also if violent

- Dicourage acting out, make it clear that he or she will be held responsible for his or her actions

- When you have to communicate your decision do it in a clear and simple way

Table 4.6 Patient–therapist relationship variables. Reproduced with permission from Elsevier

- Try to make procedures as flexible as possible

- If possible prioritize patient's requests

- Show empathy and talk about the negative aspects of present situation ('I understand that this is not good period for you; it seems to me that you feel bad, you look afraid of something')

- Engage a therapeutic alliance ('In such a difficult suituation you need help; allow me to help you')

- Don't lie or betray the patient's trust

- Do not challenge the patient, do not be confrontational, do not look the patient in the eyes

- Offer your help to discuss therapeutic aspects of mental disorder

- Give help for problem solving, especially with low copers, give alternatives to violent behaviour

- Evaluate the presence of acute and chronic stressors, especially if active, as violence triggers and related to past violence and victimization

- Give reassurance for present or past paranoid features

- Be careful with gender issues

- If needed, give an opportunity for a time out, offer food and beverage, and, if possible, allow the patient to smoke a cigarette or to phone call

In terms of medication, in the absence of contraindications the following drugs may be considered in the following order[1]:
- :Q: Rapid tranquillization—a benzodiazepine such as lorazepam or diazepam, at a small dosage, may be used. A survey by Pilowsky et al. (1992)[2] suggested that intravenous sedation with diazepam with or without haloperidol is effective. If both are administered, spacing between doses needs to be maintained.
- Typical antipsychotic drugs—there is good evidence that low-dose haloperidol (particularly intramuscularly) tends to be effective[3,4]. A single intramuscular dose of zuclopenthixol acetate (Acuphase) may be helpful in non-cooperative patients, as the effect may last up to 3 days. However, the decision to administer the latter should be carefully considered and discussed with senior clinicians.
- Atypical antipsychotic drugs—quetiapine appears to be safe and efficacious in widespread disorders such as bipolar mania[5] and Alzheimer's disease, in which it is perhaps better tolerated than haloperidol[6].
- It would be helpful to be aware of local trust policies on rapid tranquillization.

The Royal College of Psychiatrists[7] have published the algorithm shown in Fig. 4.1 as a practical example of guidelines for accident and emergency departments for the sedation of non-elderly adults.

Adults

This is given as an example of a sedation guideline for adults only, and it should not be used for young people.

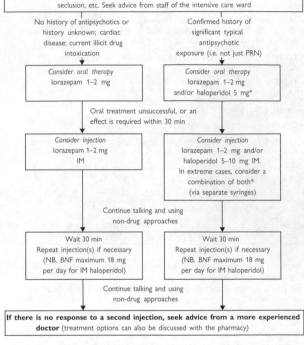

Fig. 4.1 An example of sedation guidelines for accident and emergency departments for non-elderly adults. Reproduced with kind permission from the Royal College of Psychiatrists (2004a) *Psychiatric Services to Accident and Emergency Departments.*

Notes

Ψ Combination treatment may be considered on the basis of either previous knowledge of the patient that predicts poor response to a single agent, or if the level of arousal of the patient is such that forced restraint is required and will be very difficult to repeat 30 min later.

Emergency resuscitation equipment, procyclidine injection and flumazenil injection must be available before treatment.

Monitoring of the patient must be performed and recorded according to the guidelines below after any injection is given.

Procyclidine injection 5–10 mg can be given IV or IM for acute dystonic or parkinsonian reactions.

Flumazenil (a benzodiazepine antagonist) must be given if the respiration rate falls to <10 breaths/min after lorazepam has been used (see panel below).

Give flumazenil 200 mcg IV over 15 s. If the desired level of consciousness is not obtained within 60 s, a further 100 mcg can be injected and repeated at 60 s intervals to a maximum total dose of 1 mg (1000 mcg) in 24 h (initial + eight additional doses). Monitor respiration rate continuously until it returns to baseline level.

NB. The effect of flumazenil may wear off and respiratory depression can return—monitoring must therefore continue beyond initial recovery of respiratory function.

Emergency resuscitation equipment, procyclidine injection and flumazenil injection must be available before treatment.

Example of a monitoring schedule

After injections, this monitoring schedule must be followed, unless there are compelling reasons for doing otherwise, and must be recorded in all cases:

- Pulse and respiration as soon as possible after injection, then every 5 min fo 1 h
- Temperature (using Tempadots) as soon as possilble after injection as a baseline, then at 5, 10, 15, and 60 min
- Blood pressure at 30 and 60 min after injection
- Monitor for signs of neurological reactions (e.g. acute dystonia, acute parkinsonism). If not followed, the 'responsible nurse' must document the reasons why.

Fig. 4.1 (Contd.)

References

1 Rocca P, Villari V, Bogetto F (2006). Managing the aggressive and violent patient in the psychiatric emergency. *Progress in Neuro-Psychopharmacology and Biological Psychiatry* **30**: 586–98.

2 Pilowsky LS, Ring H, Shine PJ, Battersby M, Lader M (1992). Rapid tranquillisation. A survey of emergency prescribing in a general psychiatric hospital. *British Journal of Psychiatry* **160**: 831–5.

3 Allen MH (2000). Managing the agitated psychotic patient: a reappraisal of the evidence. *Journal of Clinical Psychiatry* **61**(Suppl. 14): S1–20.

4 Baldessarini RJ, Cohen MB, Teicher MH (1988). Significance of neuroleptic dose and plasma level in the pharmacological treatment of psychoses. *Archives of General Psychiatry* **45**: 79–91.

5 Hatim A, Habil H, Jesjeet SG et al. (2006). Safety and efficacy of rapid dose administration of quetiapine in bipolar mania. *Human Psychopharmacology* **21**: 313–18.

6 Savaskan E, Schnitzler C, Schroder C et al. (2006). Treatment of behavioural, cognitive and circadian rest-activity cycle disturbances in Alzheimer's disease: haloperidol vs. quetiapine. *International Journal of Neuropsychopharmacology* (in press).

7 Royal College of Psychiatrists (2004a). *Psychiatric Services to Accident and Emergency Departments.* Council Report CR118. Royal College of Psychiatrists: London.

☺ Summary of management of aggression and violence

1. Ensure sufficient staff are present. Request police attendance if required. Disarm weapons.
2. Verbal talkdown, e.g. for half an hour—May not work if psychotic or organic.
3. Physical restraint/seclusion, e.g. for drug-free evaluation.
4. Treat psychiatric illnesses appropriately.
5. Medication as emergency:
   a. Neuroleptic antipsychotics in sedative doses
   • Best wish psychotic
   • Caution—if brain damage as increased side-effects, can worsen behaviour control, and cause akathisia, which can be misdiagnosed as agitation
   • Risk of death when high doses and high arousal.
   b. Benzodiazepines
   • Combination with neuroleptics, e.g. lorazepam/clonazepam + haloperidol
   • Risk of confusion and disinhibition of violence, especially at high doses and in brain damage
   • Spacing between doses reduces such risks
6. Staff debriefing following serious untoward incident.
   Details of the clinical situation and all interventions must be recorded in pateint's medical notes.

Emergency resuscitation equipment, procyclidine injection and flumazenil injection must be available before treatment.
Note the Mental Health Act 1983 status of the patient.

Example of a monitoring schedule
After injections, this monitoring schedule must be followed, unless there are compelling reasons for doing otherwise, and must be recorded in all cases:

• Pulse and respiration as soon as possible after injection, then every 5 min fo 1 h
• Temperature (using Tempadots) as soon as possible after injection as a baseline, then at 5, 10, 15, and 60 min
• Blood pressure at 30 and 60 min after injection
• Monitor for signs of neurological reactions (e.g. acute dystonia, acute parkinsonism).
   If not followed, the 'responsible nurse' must document the reasons why.
• Community meeting to reassure patients.
• Carers may also have to be reassured.
7. In inpatient settings it is good practice to offer patients the opportunity to document their account of the violent episode and its management, in the medical records/case notes.
8. Medication in longer-term
   a. Anticonvulsants, e.g. Carbamazepine, Valproate, and Clonazepam

- Used especially if abnormal EEG
- General slowing on EEG predicts good response if failed on neuroleptics

b. Beta-blockers, e.g. propranolol
- Often in high doses
- Especially for sudden onset severe aggression
- Beware bradycardia and hypotension

c. Lithium
- Best in bipolar disorder and recurrent irritability

d. Antidepressives
- Especially for aggression associated with affective disorder
- Especially selective serotonin reuptake inhibitors

e. Low-dose neuroleptics
- Flupenthixol (Depixol) IM

9. Cognitive behavioural approaches
   - Anger management
   - Time out
   - Token economy
   - Assertive training
   - Social skills training

10. Long-term psychotherapy.

① Safety in outpatient settings

The Royal College of Psychiatrists[1] recommend several safety precautions be taken when seeing psychiatric patients in outpatient settings:

- Recognize that the outpatient interview can be very stressful for the patient
- If the patient has been kept waiting, offer an apology
- If a patient appears to be highly aroused, decide whether the interview should take place or be postponed; if the former, then ensure the interview room has adequate safety features and try to see the patient with a colleague
- Try to use a room which:
  - Has a functioning and inconspicuous panic alarm system
  - Is close to other previously alerted staff
  - Has a door with an easy exit arrangement
  - Has a door which cannot easily be blocked
- Place yourself between the door and the patient
- Consider introducing emergency codes or phrases which alert other staff to a problem but which do not raise the alarm unduly to other patients who may be on the premises or warn the aggressor that help has been requested.

Reference

1 Royal College of Psychiatrists (2006). *Safety for Psychiatrists*. Council Report CR134. Royal College of Psychiatrists: London.

① Safety in the community

The Royal College of Psychiatrists[1] recommends several safety precautions be taken when seeing psychiatric patients in the community:

- Check your own health regularly
  - Ensure you are immunized for tetanus, tuberculosis, hepatitis B, and influenza
  - If you are pregnant or disabled, consider carefully your potential vulnerability when visiting a patient at home
- Be aware of your own limitations and experience
- Obtain as much information as possible beforehand about the patient, their carers, and even their pets
- Enquire about risky environments such as dark alleys and waste grounds; if violence is anticipated, the police may be of help in providing information
- Avoid displaying vehicle 'on-call' stickers or any other identification that show that a vehicle belongs to a healthcare professional, and conceal any bags or equipment left in the vehicle
- Carry a means of identification
- Preferably arrange joint visits with another colleague; never make night visits alone
- Respect cultural expectations
- Carry a functioning mobile telephone and programme it to access your base with one press of a button
- Ensure the staff at your base know whom you will be visiting and when you are expected to return
- After ringing the door bell, stand back from the door and stand sideways to present a narrower target
- Be prepared to abort a visit until adequate safeguards can be put in place (e.g. if a patient threatens violence)
- Make a mental note of the environment and possible routes of escape, and try to place yourself between the patient and the exit door
- Respect privacy and personal space, communicate clearly about your task, and speak courteously, with sensitivity to issues of personal dignity
- Do not wear an expensive watch or expensive jewellery—earrings, bracelets, necklaces, and ties can be used to strangle or injure
- Do not use apparently innocuous items which can be used as weapons, such as fountain pens with steel nibs
- Keep a first-aid kit in your vehicle
- Use a taxi if visiting a known problem dwelling where personal property may be at risk
- Control and restraint techniques should not be used if you are working alone, although breakaway techniques are valuable to avoid serious injury—these skills should be regularly updated.

In addition, do not interview the patient in their kitchen or in any other room where knives or other potential weapons are present.

Reference

1 Royal College of Psychiatrists (2006). *Safety for Psychiatrists*. Council Report CR134. Royal College of Psychiatrists: London.

☠ Burns

There is a small but finite risk that, as a doctor who deals with aggressive and violent patients, you might be the first medically qualified person who has to deal with victims of burns. Assess the burn size and depth, which allows calculation of fluid requirements. Use the Lund and Browder charts[1], as shown in Fig. 4.2. All major burns (>25% partial thickness in adults or >20% in children) should be transferred, with simple saline or petroleum jelly gauze dressings or even cling film, following resuscitation to a specialist burns unit.

Note that you should *not* apply cold water to large burnt areas for prolonged periods as this may worsen shock. Intravenous morphine may be titrated for analgesia.

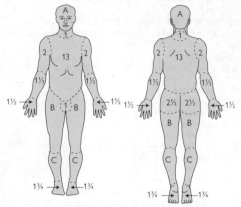

Relative percentage of body surface area affected by growth

Area	Age 0	1	5	10	15	Adult
A: half of head	9½	8½	6½	5½	4½	3½
B: half of thigh	2¾	3¼	4	4¼	4½	4¾
C: half of leg	2½	2½	2¾	3	3¼	3½

Fig. 4.2 Lund and Browder charts. Reproduced with kind permission from Longmore M *et al.* (2007). *Oxford Handbook of Clinical Medicine*, 7th edn. Oxford: Oxford University Press.

Reference

1 Longmore M, Wilkinson I, Turmezei T, Cheung CK (2007). *Oxford Handbook of Clinical Medicine*, 7th edn. Oxford University Press: Oxford.

Victims of abuse, violence, and disaster

Non-accidental injury of children 88
Consequences for adult functioning of childhood
    sexual abuse 89
Child abduction 89
Spouse abuse (replaces term wife-battering)/
    intimate partner violence 90
Elder abuse 92
Morbid jealousy (Othello syndrome) 94
Erotomania (de Clérambault's syndrome) 96
Stalking 96
Rape and sexual assault of women 98
Rape and sexual assault of men 100
Post-traumatic stress disorder 102
Acute stress reaction 108
Adjustment disorder 108

Victimization is associated with mental disorder. For instance, the victims of childhood abuse and neglect develop an excess of psychological sequelae, including post traumatic stress disorder (PTSD), and may become offenders, including paedophile offenders, in later life; i.e. the abused becoming the abuser (psychological identification with the aggressor). In turn, offending itself can lead to secondary victimization; the prevention, amelioration, and treatment of victimization is therefore important.

☠ Non-accidental injury of children

This term has replaced that of 'baby bashing', coined by Kempe and Kempe[1] in 1961 as an emotive term to highlight the problem.

Characteristic features of different members of the families in which non-accidental injury of children occurs are as follows.

Children
- Usually less than 3 years of age
- Failure to thrive
- Persistent crying
- Multiple injuries in time and space
- Delay in reporting and contradictory histories of injuries.

Parents
- Often abused themselves and unhappy children
- Lower social class families
- Isolated and no support
- Marital disharmony
- Unwanted pregnancy
- No contraception.

Mother
- Often teenager, unmarried, neurotic, and/or learning disability
- Expects love from child
- Not infrequently on diazepam (valium).

Father
- In about half the cases, not biological father
- Two-thirds are not married
- Often has personality disorder
- Criminal in two-thirds of cases and one in three has conviction for violence
- Beats wife in a quarter of cases
- Competes with the child, whom he rejects, for his wife/partner's attention.

The incidence of psychosis in parents is low, but may be higher in severely abused cases. In the UK there are 80 child murders a year; 60 of whom are killed by their parents and 10 by strangers.

Note that filicide is the killing of one's son or daughter.

Matricide is most often committed by individuals suffering with schizophrenia.

Reference
1 Kempe CH, Kempe RS (1978). *Child Abuse*. Fontana Books: London.

Consequences for adult functioning of childhood sexual abuse

- Personality difficulties
- Anxiety
- Depression
- Sexual adjustment difficulties
- Substance abuse
- Decreased socioeconomic status because of disruption of sense of effective agency and low self-esteem
- Intergenerational: uncaring or over-controlling parenting.

⊙ Child abduction

The relevant law is the Child Abduction Act 1984. There are three main groups:
1. Abduction by parents, usually in custody disputes
2. Abduction of older children, usually by a man with a sexual motive[1]
3. Baby stealing, the least common group, usually carried out by women.

In the UK in Victorian times children were stolen to obtain their clothes. When women steal babies, in general the babies are well cared for and usually quickly recovered.

Categories of baby stealing

As described by d'Orbán[2] these include:
1. Comforting offences, e.g. those with learning disability who steal a baby to play with or for comfort.
2. Manipulative offences, where the motive may be an attempt to influence a man with whom her relationship is insecure by presenting the baby to their partner pretending the child is his, e.g. following a miscarriage of a pregnancy by him or threatened desertion.
3. Psychotic offences where offences are motivated by delusional ideas, e.g. that the child is a Messiah.

Reference

1 D'Orbán PT, Haydn-Smith P (1985). Men who steal children. *British Medical Journal* **290**: 1784.
2 D'Orbán PT (1976). Child stealing: a typology of female offenders. *British Journal of Criminology* **16**: 275–81.

⚠ Spouse abuse (replaces term wife-battering)/intimate partner violence

The true incidence is obscured by the hidden nature of the behaviour and problems in definition, e.g. over the degree of violence. This category is responsible in England and Wales for 16% of all violent crimes, and results in two homicides of women a week, with 40% killed in the bedroom or kitchen. It is often associated with psychological abuse and behaviour such as excessive jealousy and control of money. In the USA it has been estimated that in 25–30% of marriages one partner would push, shove or grab the other at some point. Punches and kicks occurred in 13% of marriages, and beating up or using a weapon in 5% of marriages. Surveys show that while wives attack their husbands at a not substantially lesser frequency, such attacks are much less violent and usually defensive.

Male abusers are often inarticulate, demanding, and find violence empowering. Typologies include those with a frequent loss of temper and those who undertake cold deliberate assaults, as well as over-controlled individuals who 'snap'. Jealousy within the relationship is a factor noted in two-thirds of cases. Half of all offenders have been exposed to domestic violence as a child, and 50% of assaults follow alcohol abuse. Wife-battering has also been associated with gambling, unemployment, and an otherwise criminal record. Offenders are often remorseful following violence. Women may be trapped in violent marriages economically, owing to a lack of alternative housing or because of feelings of responsibility for children and/or by learned helplessness.

Battered women syndrome

This has been described as being characterized by:
- Depression
- Loss of self-esteem
- Post-traumatic stress disorder
- Substance abuse
- Suicidality
- Physical health problems
- Sexual problems.

Intimate partner abuse

This mainly affects women (wives, girlfriends, female partners). If intimate partner (spouse) abuse is suspected, it can be difficult to persuade the female victim to admit that she has been physically and mentally abused. A recent Canadian screening randomized trial has found that women prefer self-completed questionnaire approaches to face-to-face questioning[1]. Assessment of the victim must be carried out with great sensitivity. Check that the victim is not suicidal or depressed, and that she is not abusing alcohol or drugs or suffering from an anxiety disorder.

Management

The management can be difficult, particularly if the victim denies the abuse and insists on returning to her abusive partner. If there is a high risk of the abuse continuing, social services may need to be involved and the police may need to be informed. If the risk is lower, and the victim and her partner agree, then marital therapy may be arranged.

- Voluntary refuges are now widely available
- Anger management techniques can be applied to offenders
- A non-molestation injunction can also be sought, including attached power of arrest
- New multidisciplinary case conference management approach (MARAC) is developing in the UK.

Reference

1 MacMillan HL, Wathen N, Jamieson E et al. (2006). *Journal of the American Medical Association* **296**: 530–6.

⚙ Elder abuse

Estimates have been made that up to 500 000 older people are abused each day in the UK. Elder abuse includes violence, neglect or emotional abuse of elderly relatives, often a surviving widowed elderly mother. The term replaces the term 'Granny bashing' (coined by Renvoize in 1978 in *Web of Violence*[1]). The offender is often a son or daughter (50% over 60 years of age) of the victim and lives together with the victim. The British prevalence rate is between 1.5 and 5.6%. Abused elders are no more physically or mentally infirm than non-abused elders.

The abuser may be otherwise under stress from marital or financial problems, be depressed, have a history of substance misuse and/or personal history of being abused themselves, and be unable to cope with the added stress of looking after the victim who may be emotionally and economically dependent. Unresolved emotional conflict is often present.

There is often a history of families being reluctant to take over the care of elder relatives but being under pressure to do so. The situation occasionally arises owing to an equally aged spouse having to cope with/care for the victim. Emotional conflict may be present between the abuser and abused. Unqualified staff in poorly managed nursing homes may also abuse the elderly.

Victim vulnerability factors, e.g. disability, dementia or paranoid illness, may be present.

NB. Most violence is within the family as this is where individuals are most physically and emotionally close to others.

Reference

1 Renvoize J (1978). *Web of Violence*. Routledge, Kegan Paul: London.

☼ Morbid jealousy (Othello syndrome)

Delusions of infidelity about a sexual partner which can lead the sufferer to examine underwear, sexual organs of partner, etc. In an attempt to find proof of unfaithfulness and, on occasions, attempt to extract confessions by violence. This not infrequently leads to severe aggression towards and the killing of the sexual partner about whom the delusions are held. Occurs in men over six times more commonly than in women (compare with erotomania which is more frequent in women). This condition usually commences in the 40s after about 10 years of marriage/relationship, and is present for about 4 years before presenting. Responsible for 12% of homicides due to mental illness[1].

Aetiology

Morbid jealousy is associated with alcoholism, schizophrenia, and delusional disorder. It may be a forerunner of a later schizophrenic illness, this only manifesting after serious violence. It is also associated with impotence in men. Psychodynamic theories of aetiology postulate that the suspicious attitudes may be a projection of the individual's own desires for infidelity on to the victim-partner or a more internally acceptable, unconscious manifestation of repressed homosexuality. Morbid jealousy is often associated with low self-esteem, with resulting feelings of insecurity that the partner may not really love him and may wish to leave him for someone else.

Management

This is often difficult because of the lack of insight of the subject, and the sexual partner's belief that they can overcome their spouse's unjustifiable beliefs. Underlying psychiatric conditions should be adequately treated. Individuals should stop any alcohol abuse. Antipsychotic medication may help if compliance can be obtained. Separation may be the only answer and there is a risk of recurrence in future relationships, e.g. case of Iliffe who killed four wives in spite of having spent periods in Broadmoor hospital. It is best to work with a co-therapist, e.g. a social worker, who remains involved with the spouse, advising her of refuges, etc. while the psychiatrist concentrates on the patient.

NB. Rivalry is where two individuals are in competition for the same object. No aggression to object.

Envy is where one individual desires someone or something that belongs to someone else. Aggression to competitor or self but not to object.

Jealousy involves fantasies of losing the object to a rival. Aggression is directed not to the rival but to the object, i.e. spouse. All through history and across cultures, the main cause of female homicide is male jealousy.

Jealousy can be normal or excessive (sometimes even in the absence of delusions); this is also termed morbid, i.e. for neurotic, obsessional or delusional reasons, including being secondary to affective disorder. It also arises in paranoid personalities. The boundary between normal and pathological jealousy may be indistinct. However, psychotic jealousy often responds better to treatment than neurotic jealousy.

NB. Delusional jealousy can develop even when the spouse has, in fact, been unfaithful. The way the delusional belief develops may be more diagnostic than pure content of the belief. (NB. Philosophical criticism: a statement of fact cannot be derived from a statement of value?)

Reference

1 Mowat R (1966). *Morbid Jealousy and Murder*. Tavistock: London.

! Erotomania (de Clérambault's syndrome)

This is a delusional disorder that another person, often unobtainable and of higher social status, loves the patient (usually female) intensely. It may be primary or secondary due to a paranoid or affective disorder. It is usually associated with paranoid psychosis or schizophrenia rather than a pure monodelusional disorder. Only in some cases will there be disruptive antisocial behaviour, e.g. phone calls, letter writing, following the victim, but repeated rebuttals may lead to hatred and dangerous behaviour. Dangerousness is increased if there is a history of multiple delusional objects in the past and premorbid antisocial personality[1].

Reference
1 Menzies RP, Fedoroff JP, Green CM, Isaacson K (1995). Prediction of dangerous behaviour in male erotomania. *British Journal of Psychiatry* **166**: 529–36.

Stalking

This is the wilful, malicious, and repeated following and harassing of another person. The term originated in relation to celebrities in California in the late 1980s, but 90% of stalking follows the breakdown of a relationship.

Classification (after Mullen et al., 2000)[1]
- Rejected stalker—mixture of revenge and desire for reconciliation
- Intimacy seeking—includes deluded
- Incompetent stalker/suitor—lacks social skills; may be intellectually limited
- Resentful stalker—intends to cause fear
- Predatory stalker—prior to, or fantasies about, sexual assault.

NB. False victim—may, in fact, be the stalker.

Risk of violence
Violence is threatened in 50% of cases. The homicide rate is 2%, but nine out of ten domestic homicides are stalked before murder.

Risk of post-traumatic stress disorder
This has been estimated to be 37%[1]. The risk rises to 55% if absence of one overwhelming stressor is taken into account.

Management
Prevention may be most important.
Protection from Harassment Act 1997 in England and Wales (injunction and criminal sentence).

Reference
1 Mullen PE, Pathe M, Purcell R (2000). *Stalkers and their Victims*. Cambridge University Press: Cambridge.

☠ Rape and sexual assault of women

It is not usually the duty of a psychiatrist to deal directly with rape or sexual assault in the emergency setting. However, if you do encounter a case of alleged rape or sexual assault, it is helpful to be aware of the advice given to doctors working in accident and emergency departments.

Although by definition a sexual offence, the rape of a woman often represents an act of displaced aggression by the perpetrator, who enjoys the domination and denigration, and often perceives passivity in a victim (often induced by fear) as consent. At least 30% of victims are acquaintances of the perpetrator.

It may also be important, if one is in the position of being the first point of referral, to facilitate further referral for appropriate management.

Rape and sexual assault are considered grossly under-reported. Victims may present with blunt or penetrating genital injuries and give misleading histories. A full examination is required. Penetrating injuries may be caused by assault, foreign body insertion, or intrauterine contraceptive device (IUCD) injuries. Sometimes, female victims initially decline examination but later agree, whereupon examination can still yield useful information.

Occasionally female victims telephone emergency departments for advice after rape. They should be advised to inform the police immediately and then attend a police station or the emergency department and avoid changing their clothes, washing, cleaning their teeth, and going to the toilet.

Requirements for interview and examination

Interview and examination must be handled sensitively and professionally. Requirements include:
- A specially equipped room and a female member of staff present
- Documentation must be meticulous and legible
- Established protocols to ensure that such incidents are investigated and treated are now widely available
- Emergency department staff perform emergency treatment and resuscitation of life-threatening and serious injuries
- Otherwise forensic physicians/police surgeons, on occasion with gynaecologists, deal with all other aspects, including collection of evidence.

History

- Circumstances and time of assault
- Contraceptive history
- Sexual history
- Date of last period
- Pregnant?

Examination

- Vaginal, oral or anal injuries
- Record other injuries, e.g. bites, bruises
- Police can usefully photograph injuries with the individual's consent.

Investigations
- Obtain written consent
- Retain clothing, loose hairs, finger nail clippings, tampons
- Swab vaginal, oral, and anal areas
- Pregnancy test
- Take blood for future DNA testing.

Treatment
- Emergency resuscitation
- Refer urgently significant genital injuries for operative treatment
- Consider postcoital contraception and prophylactic treatment against hepatitis C, HIV, and tetanus
- Arrange STD/GUM (sexually transmitted disease/genitourinary medicine) clinic follow-up appointment following prophylactic antibiotic medication, if considered appropriate
- Initial supportive counselling and safe place to stay (social services may assist)
- Arrange further counselling, e.g. from independent rape crisis centre.

Counselling of a victim may have to address problems of guilt, pregnancy, sexually transmitted infections (STI or VD—venereal disease), shunning by friends, and court appearances. The more a victim struggled, the more likely she is to sustain injuries (which is in contrast to non-sexual violent offences). However, the less the victim struggles, the more likely it is that guilt and depression result.

☠ Rape and sexual assault of men

Male rape did not exist as an offence until the legal definition was changed in November 1994[1]. Male rape is generally recognized as being under-reported; according to the Home Office, in the UK it has increased from 150 cases in 1995 to 852 in 2002–2003, with 4096 recorded incidents of indecent assault of males in 2002–2003[2], although the Home Office has stated that these figures are unlikely to reflect the real experiences of such crimes. According to the general practice cross-sectional survey by Coxell and colleagues (1999)[3], of 2474 men attending one of 18 general practices, almost 3% of men in England report non-consensual sexual experiences as adults; non-consensual sexual experiences are associated with a greater prevalence of psychological problems, alcohol misuse, and self-harm.

The rape and sexual assault of men and women have been compared in studies of the characteristics of those attending St Mary's Sexual Assault Referral Centre, Greater Manchester in England, UK.[4,5] This centre opened in October 1986. Up to May 2003 it had seen 376 male (370 individual clients) and 7789 female cases (7403 clients). Of these, significantly fewer males reported to the police than females, although this difference disappeared after 2003. Of the male cases who underwent a forensic medical examination, 18% presented with an anal injury, which was significantly more than in the female victims; however, significantly fewer males than females were found to have sustained injuries to other body areas. (There were no significant differences between the sexes for age of the client, and presence in the assault of weapons or additional violence.)

Another important study of male victims of sexual assault was published by Reeves and colleagues (2004).[1] This was based on 92 males undergoing forensic examination between 2000 and 2003 at the Haven, a specialist centre for the management of sexual assault in south London. The men were aged from 12 to 51 years, with most (83%) being aged from 12 to 35 years. Of the men involved, 89% were sexually active, and of these 30% were heterosexual and 34% homosexual, while the remainder provided no information regarding sexual orientation. Most (86%) were referred by the police. There was an increased vulnerability to assault noted in many of the victims, including alcohol misuse, drug misuse, and mental health difficulties. When known, while the assailant was usually one person (66% of cases), in 28% of cases two or more assailants were involved; in 4% of cases the assailants were reported as being women. The sexual assault was frequently accompanied by other physical assault, and in 20% of cases there was the use or threat of use of a weapon by the assailant(s). Rape (non-consensual receptive anal intercourse) or attempted rape was reported in 64% of cases and was the most common assault. Non-genital injuries were documented in 40%. Anal injuries were seen in 34%. Condom use by the assailants was reported in only two cases.

A good psychosexual history is an essential aspect of any assessment in psychiatry; in these cases, it would be required to be more comprehensive. Based on these studies, it is reasonable to adopt a low threshold to enquire about being the victim of rape or attempted rape in a male patient who gives any indication of having been sexually assaulted—for example, if anal injuries are present. Patients living in all-male environments, such as prisons, may also be at increased risk and should be asked directly about sexual assault. Enquiries should be made about alcohol misuse, drug misuse, suicidal thoughts, and other mental health problems. If there is any history of sexual assault, then there is clearly a risk of sexually transmitted infection, including HIV, and consent should be obtained from the patient to test him for such an infection and subsequently to treat him as necessary.

If abuse is suspected, and particularly if it involves minors, it may be necessary to involve social services. In cases involving minors, it may be necessary to inform the appropriate child protection named consultant/nurse for the Trust.

References

1 Reeves I, Jawad R, Welch J (2004). Risk of undiagnosed infection in men attending a sexual assault referral centre. *Sexually Transmitted Infections* **80**: 524–5.
2 Home Office (2003). *The British Crime Survey*. Home Office Publications: London.
3 Coxell A, King M, Mezey G, Gordon D (1999). Lifetime prevalence, characteristics and associated problems of non-consensual sex in men: cross-sectional survey. *British Medical Journal* **318**: 846–50.
4 McLean IA, Balding V, White C (2004). Forensic medical aspects of male-on-male rape and sexual assault in greater Manchester. *Medicine, Science and the Law* **44**: 165–9.
5 McLean IA, Balding V, White C (2005). Further aspects of male-on-male rape and sexual assault in greater Manchester. *Medicine, Science and the Law* **45**: 225–32.

⊙ Post-traumatic stress disorder

Victims of traumatic events may suffer from post-traumatic stress disorder. Rarely, this may present as an emergency. It is important to bear in mind that those looking after emergency cases, including medical and nursing staff, may also be affected by post-traumatic stress disorder.

This is a common reaction of normal individuals to an extreme trauma likely to cause pervasive stress to anyone. Although predisposing factors such as personality traits and previous history of neurotic illness may lower the threshold for the development of a syndrome or aggravate the course, they are neither sufficient nor necessary. The condition is seen as arising from the overwhelming of and overloading of normal emotional processing.

Diagnosis

The ICD-10[1] states that post-traumatic stress disorder (F43.1):

> '...arises as a delayed and/or protracted response to a stressful event or situation (either short- or long-lasting) of an exceptionally threatening or catastrophic nature, which is likely to cause pervasive distress in almost anyone...'

Examples of such traumatic events given by ICD-10 include:
- Natural disaster
- Man-made disaster
- Combat
- Serious accident
- Witnessing the violent death of others
- Being the victim of torture
- Being the victim of terrorism
- Being the victim of rape or other crime.

Other examples of causes described include:
- Hospitalization
- Detention under the Mental Health Act
- Psychotic symptoms
- Offending.

It is important to realize that victims of post-traumatic stress disorder often do not admit to symptoms, e.g. flashbacks, nightmares, unless directly asked. A high level of clinical suspicion is therefore required.

According to the ICD-10 diagnostic system of assessment,

> Typical symptoms include episodes of repeated reliving of the trauma in intrusive memories ('flashbacks') or dreams, occurring against the persisting background of a sense of 'numbness' and emotional blunting, detachment from other people, unresponsiveness to surroundings, anhedonia, and avoidance of activities and situations reminiscent of the trauma. Commonly there is fear and avoidance of cues that remind the sufferer of the original trauma. Rarely, there may be dramatic, acute bursts of fear, panic or aggression, triggered by stimuli arousing a sudden recollection and/or re-enactment of the trauma or of the original reaction to it.

There is usually a state of autonomic hyperarousal with hypervigilance, an enhanced startle reaction, and insomnia. Anxiety and depression are commonly associated with the above symptoms and signs, and suicidal ideation is not infrequent. Excessive use of alcohol or drugs may be a complicating factor.

The onset follows the trauma with a latency of a few weeks to months, but not more than 6 months, and the condition must last for at least a month.

The diagnostic criteria for post-traumatic stress disorder in DSM-IV-TR,[2] in which it is named post-traumatic stress disorder (309.81) are summarized in Table 5.1.

Table 5.1 Diagnostic criteria for 309.81 post-traumatic stress disorder

A. The person has been exposed to a traumatic event in which both of the following were present:

1. The person experienced, witnessed, or was confronted with an event or events that involved actual or threatened death or serious injury, or a threat to the physical integrity of self or others.

2. The person's response involved intense fear, helplessness, or horror. **NB.**: In children, this may be expressed instead by disorganized or agitated behaviour

B. The traumatic event is persistently re-experienced in one (or more) of the following ways:

1. Recurrent disstressing recollections of the event, including images, thoughts, or preceptions. **NB.**: In children this may be expressed in repetitive play.

2. Recurrent disstressing dreams of the event. **NB.**: In children, these may be frightening dreams without recognizable contents.

3. Acting or feeling as if the truamatic event were recurring (includes a sense of reliving the experience, illusions, hallucinastions, and dissociative flashback episodes, including those that occur on awakening or when intoxicated).

4. Intense psychological distress at and psychological reactivity on exposure to internal or external cues that symbolize or resemble an aspect of the traumatic event.

C. Persistent avoidance of stimuli associated with the trauma and numbing of general responsiveness (not present before the trauma), as indicated by three (or more) of the following:

1. Efforts to avoid thoughts, feeling or conversations associated with the trauma.

2. Efforts to avoid activities, places, or people that arouse recollections of the trauma.

3. Inablility to recall important aspects of the trauma.

4. Markedly diminished interest or participation in significant activities.

5. Feeling of detachment or estrangemant from others.

6. Restricted range of affect (e.g. unable to have loving feelings).

7. Sense of a foreshortened future.

Table 5.1 (*Contd.*)

D. Persistant symptoms of increased arousal (not present before the trauma), as indicated by two (or more) of the following:

1. Difficulty falling or staying asleep.
2. Irritabilty or outbursts of anger.
3. Difficulty concentrating.
4. Hypervigilance.
5. Exaggerated startle response.

E.   Duration of the disturbance is more than 1 month

F.   The disturbance causes clinically significant distress or impairment in social, occupastional, or important areas of functioning.

Specify if:

Acute: if duration of symptoms is less than 3 months

Chronic: if duration of symptoms is 3 months or more

Specify if:

With delayed onset: if onset of symptoms is at least 6 months after the stress

Robert Spitzer helped to introduce post-traumatic stress disorder into DSM-III[3] and helped to modify the criteria several years later for DSM-III-R[4,5]. However, there have been criticisms of these criteria, and, partly in order to help reduce the rate of false positives, Spitzer and colleagues (2007) have proposed a revised criteria for post-traumatic stress disorder for DSM-V (Table 5.2) (which has not been published at the time of writing):

Other traumatic events and vulnerability factors

Many traumatic causes have been given above in the sections on ICD-10 and the DSM. It is worth considering several aspects in a little more detail.

Terrorism is, sadly, a phenomenon with which we are increasingly required to be familiar. Post-traumatic stress disorder can follow savage acts of terrorism, even if the exposure to such acts has been purely indirect, via the media (particularly television and the internet). Following acts of terrorism, or widespread media coverage of such acts, there needs to be a heightened awareness of the possibility of people suffering from post-traumatic stress disorder. At the time of writing, the most extreme act of terrorism was that of 9/11, which took place on 11th September 2001. Saylor et al. (2006)[6] found that among American university students who had indirectly experienced this act via the media, those with previous exposure to crime had significantly more post-traumatic stress disorder symptoms related to 9/11 exposure. High crime stress level has previously been found to be significantly associated with post-traumatic stress disorder following the crime, where high crime stress is defined as crime that includes perceived life threat, actual injury, or completed rape[7].

Table 5.2 Revised criteria for post-traumatic stress disorder for DSM-V

A. The person has been exposed to a traumatic event in which both of the following were present:

1. The person *directly* experienced or witnessed an event or events that involved actual or threatened death or serious injury, or a threat to the physical integrity of self or others.
2. The person's response involved intense fear, helplessness, or horror. NB. In children, this may be expressed instead by disorganized or agitated behaviour.

B. The traumatic event is persistently re-experienced in one (or more) of the following ways:

1. Recurrent and intrusive distressing recollections of the event, including images, thoughts, or perceptions. NB. In young children, repetitive play may occur in which themes or aspects of the trauma are expressed.
2. Recurrent distressing dreams of the event. NB. In children, there may be frightening dreams without recognizable content.
3. Acting or feeling as if the traumatic event were recurring (includes a sense of reliving the experience, illusions, hallucinations, and dissociative flashback episodes, including those that occur on awakening or when intoxicated). NB. In young children, trauma-specific re-enactment may occur.
4. Intense psychological distress at exposure to internal or external cues that symbolize or resemble an aspect of the traumatic event.
5. Physiological reactivity on exposure to internal or external cues that symbolize or resemble an aspect of the traumatic event.

C. *Four* (or more) of the following:

1. Efforts to avoid thoughts, feelings, or conversations associated with the trauma.
2. Efforts to avoid activities, places, or people that arouse recollections of the trauma.
3. Feeling of detachment or estrangement from others.
4. Restricted range of affect (e.g. unable to have loving feelings).
5. Sense of a foreshortened future (e.g. *unrealistic fears of not having* a career, marriage, children, or a normal life span *because of one's future being cut short*).
6. Hypervigilance.
7. Exaggerated startle response.

D. Duration of the disturbance (symptoms in Criteria B and C) is more than 1 month.

E. Either (1) or (2):

1. The symptoms develop within a week of the event.
2. If delayed onset, the onset of symptoms is associated with an event that is thematically related to the trauma itself (e.g. onset of symptoms in a rape survivor when initiating a sexual relationship).

F. The disturbance causes clinically significant distress or impairment in social, occupational, or other important areas of functioning.

G. Not due to an exacerbation of a pre-existing mood, anxiety, or personality disorder or to malingering.

As alluded to above, alcohol dependence and post traumatic stress disorder often show comorbidity. Those with a history of childhood trauma may be particularly vulnerable to relapse following treatment for alcohol dependence[8].

Medical and paramedical staff in stressful work environments may suffer an increased risk of developing post-traumatic stress disorder. For example, intensive care unit nursing staff have been found to have an increased prevalence of post-traumatic stress disorder symptoms when compared to other general nurses[9].

Major outbreaks of pandemic infections can also be expected to cause post-traumatic stress disorder symptoms in front-line medical staff. At the time of writing, a major influenza pandemic has been predicted to strike. A recent example of what might be expected is furnished by the far less severe outbreak of SARS (severe acute respiratory syndrome) in 2003, which affected 29 countries and was demanding on front-line medical and nursing staff, particularly in accident and emergency departments. A study from Taiwan[10] found that 94% (86 out of 92) of emergency department (high-risk) medical staff (consisting of doctors and nurses) found the SARS outbreak to be a traumatic experience, with the staff having more severe post-traumatic stress disorder symptoms than medical staff working in a lower risk psychiatric ward.

Prevention

Primary prevention has been attempted through stress inoculation in high-risk groups, e.g. exposure to dead bodies.

Secondary prevention strategies have been found to be of value in aiding early emotional processing, e.g. meetings of survivors and critical incident debriefing within 1–2 days. The efficacy of such measures is, however, unproven, and inappropriate and ill-timed interventions or interventions which lead to inappropriate rumination on the trauma can be harmful.

Management

Many cases go undetected owing to the individual's reluctance to discuss symptoms and seek help. Making the diagnosis can be reassuring to the individual, who often feels that no-one else can understand what he has been through. The route of referral may therefore vary depending on the time of exposure to the trauma, for example, at a crash scene, or years later following a war.

Management needs to include treatment of the primary problem and any associated complications such as alcohol or drug abuse.

Central to most treatment approaches is rehearsal of the 'trauma story', for example by 'testimony' or by a cognitive behavioural approach. The latter is probably the treatment of choice. This should include exposure, imaginal and/or *in vivo*, to counter avoidance and escape behaviour, and thought-identifying, evidence-gathering, and Socratic questioning, to counter the maintaining beliefs held about the self, the world, the trauma, and the future[11]. Short-term group cognitive behaviour therapy for post-traumatic stress disorder even appears to be helpful for children, as illustrated in a study following the 1999 Athens earthquake[12].

A recent systematic review and meta-analysis by Ipser et al. (2006)[13] concluded that medication can be effective in treating post-traumatic stress disorder, and supported the use of SSRIs as first-line treatment. Compared with placebo, pharmacotherapy was more effective in diminishing symptom severity, post-traumatic stress disorder-experiencing/intrusion, avoidance/numbing, hyperarousal symptom clusters, comorbid depression, and disability. Of the medication classes reviewed, evidence of treatment efficacy was most convincing for the SSRIs.

References

1 World Health Organization (1992). The ICD-10 Classification of Mental and Behavioural Disorders. Clinical Descriptions and Diagnostic Guidelines. World Health Organization: Geneva.

2 American Psychiatric Association (2000). Diagnostic and Statistical Manual of Mental Disorders, 4th edn, text revision (DSM-IV-TR). American Psychiatric Association: Washington DC.

3 American Psychiatric Association (1980). Diagnostic and Statistical Manual of Mental Disorders, 3rd edn (DSM-III). American Psychiatric Association: Washington DC.

4 American Psychiatric Association (1987). Diagnostic and Statistical Manual of Mental Disorders, 3rd edn, revised (DSM-III-R). American Psychiatric Association: Washington DC.

5 Spitzer RL, First MB, Wakefield JC (2007). Saving PTSD from itself in DSM-V. Journal of Anxiety Disorders (in press).

6 Saylor C, DeRoma V, Swickert R (2006). College students with previous exposure to crime report more PTSD after 9-11-2001. Psychological Reports 99: 581–2.

7 Resnick HS, Kilpatrick DG, Best CL, Kramer TL (1992). Vulnerability-stress factors in development of posttraumatic stress disorder. Journal of Nervous and Mental Disorders 180: 424–30.

8 Schumacher JA, Coffey SF, Stasiewicz PR (2006). Symptom severity, alcohol craving, and age of trauma onset in childhood and adolescent trauma survivors with comorbid alcohol dependence and posttraumatic stress disorder. American Journal on Addictions 15: 422–35.

9 Mealer ML, Shelton A, Berg B, Rothbaum B, Moss M (2007). Increased prevalence of post traumatic stress disorder symptoms in critical care nurses. American Journal of Respiratory and Critical Care Medicine (in press).

10 Lin C-Y, Peng Y-C, Wu Y-H et al. (2007). The psychological effect of severe acute respiratory syndrome on emergency department staff. Emergency Medicine Journal 24: 12–17.

11 Grant P, Young PR, DeRubeis RJ (2005). Cognitive and behavioral therapies. In: GO Gabbard, JS Beck and J Holmes (eds.) Oxford Textbook of Psychotherapy. Oxford University Press: Oxford.

12 Giannopoulou I, Dikaiakou A, Yule W (2006). Cognitive-behavioural group intervention for PTSD symptoms in children following the Athens 1999 earthquake: a pilot study. Clinical Child Psychology and Psychiatry 11: 543–53.

13 Ipser J, Seedat S, Stein DJ (2006). Pharmacotherapy for post-traumatic stress disorder—a systematic review and meta-analysis. South African Medical Journal 96: 1088–96.

✛ Acute stress reaction

This is more common than post-traumatic stress disorder. It is the response in apparently normal individuals to exceptional physical and/or mental stress, such as:

- Overwhelming traumatic experience involving serious threat to the individual or loved ones
- Unusually sudden and threatening change in their social position/network, e.g. multiple bereavements, domestic fire.

The risk is increased if physical exhaustion or other organic factors are present.

Individual vulnerability and coping capacity vary as not all exposed to exceptional stress develop this disorder. A mixed and usually changing clinical picture is characteristic, e.g. initial state of 'daze', followed by depression, anxiety, anger, despair, over-activity (flight reaction of fugue) or withdrawal. No one symptom predominates for long.

The condition resolves rapidly within a few hours or days upon removal from the stressful environment. If stress continues or cannot be reversed, symptoms usually begin to diminish after 24–48 h and are usually minimal after 3 days.

ⓘ Adjustment disorder

Adjustment disorders are states of emotional distress and disturbance, usually interfering with social functioning, arising in a period of adapting to a significant life change or stressful life event, such as a bereavement or separation.

- Onset within 1 month of event. Duration usually not more than 6 months.
- Individual predisposition and vulnerability more important than in an acute stress reaction, but stress necessary.
- Other predisposing factors include culture shock, grief reactions, and hospitalization in children.
- Types include brief or prolonged depressive reactions; mixed anxiety and depressive reactions; or disturbance of conduct, e.g. in adolescence.

📖 Grief and bereavement reactions are covered in Chapter 13.

Homelessness, loneliness, and isolation

Prevalence and factors associated with homelessness *110*
Housing and mental health *110*
Loneliness *111*
Psychiatric disorders in homeless people *111*
Management of homelessness *112*
Legal framework of management *113*

It is important to differentiate homelessness (not having a home) from rooflessness (sleeping rough). Among both groups, the clinician should have a high index of suspicion that such individuals may suffer from alcoholism, substance misuse, and/or schizophrenia, as well as having high rates of physical morbidity. Such individuals are also more likely to have a history of being in care and in prison. A question to consider is whether such individuals are homeless mentally ill, or mentally ill homeless.

⑦ Prevalence and factors associated with homelessness

In general, in the developed world homelessness is an increasing problem among those who suffer from psychiatric disorders. In their large 1-year (1999–2000) study of over 10 000 patients treated for schizophrenia, bipolar disorder, or major depression in the San Diego County Adult Mental Health Services, California, Folsom et al. (2005)[1] found that the prevalence of homelessness was 15%. The following factors were found to be associated with homelessness:

• Male gender
• African–American ethnicity
• The presence of a substance use disorder
• Lack of Medicaid
• A diagnosis of schizophrenia or bipolar disorder
• Poorer functioning.

Poor socio-occupational functioning, poor self-care, and poor physical health are characteristic. Homeless patients were found to use more inpatient and emergency-type services and fewer outpatient-type services.

There is an increased prevalence of schizophrenia in urban areas and among the lower social classes, which has been explained by a social drift hypothesis (such individuals drift down the social scale although their parents show normal social class distribution).

Reference

1 Folsom DP, Hawthorne W, Lindamer L, et al. (2005). Prevalence and risk factors for homelessness and utilization of mental health services among 10 340 patients with serious mental illness in a large public mental health system. American Journal of Psychiatry 162: 370–6.

Housing and mental health

Housing itself may influence mental health, e.g. through high-rise estates, overcrowding, sanitary conditions and the ecology of urban living. This is acknowledged in the UK through 'extra points' towards rehousing from housing waiting lists, although this may help little due to the demand for housing from other vulnerable groups.

Poverty is associated with mental ill health and bad housing. However, 24-hour staffed or supported accommodation, especially if linked to assertive outreach or case management programmes, can reduce time in hospital and psychiatric symptoms, and improve quality of life and housing stability.

⑦ Loneliness

The subjective experience of loneliness is a factor associated with referral for urgent psychiatric care[1]. Indeed, in 1999, Geller and colleagues[2] reported a statistically significant correlation between loneliness score and total hospital emergency department visits in the USA the level of loneliness being measured using the University of California–Los Angeles Loneliness Scale. They concluded that loneliness is a predictor of hospital emergency department use independent of chronic illness, and is potentially very expensive to society. It is also important to note that male loneliness resulting from living alone appears to be a risk factor for suicide and suicide attempts[3].

References

1 Mantrana Ridruejo L, Luque Budia A, Conde Diaz M, Dobladez Soriano S (2004). Factors associated to urgent referral in a mental health center. *Actas Españolas de Psiquiatría* **32**: 16–22.

2 Geller J, Janson P, McGovern E, Valdini A (1999). Loneliness as a predictor of hospital emergency department use. *Journal of Family Practice* **48**: 801–4.

3 Hattori T, Taketani K, Ogasawara Y (1995). Suicide and suicide attempts in general hospital psychiatry: clinical and statistical study. *Psychiatry and Clinical Neurosciences* **49**: 43–8.

① Psychiatric disorders in homeless people

Susser and colleagues (1989)[1] assessed 223 homeless men at first entry to municipal men's shelters in New York. Their findings were as follows:

> The majority of men had a history of mental disorder or of heavy substance use. On diagnostic interview, 17% of the men had a definite or probable history of psychosis, and another 8% had a possible history of psychosis. A confident diagnosis of schizophrenia was made in 8%. A history of alcohol or other drug abuse was evident in 58%. Cocaine was already (in 1985) the drug of choice; 27% of the study sample had used it more than 50 times. One-third of the men were in extreme distress, much of it apparently acute and associated with the transition to the shelter, and 7% reported suicidal thoughts at the time of the interview. The newly homeless, compared with those who had been homeless for much of the 5 years prior to shelter entry, were younger and had fewer psychiatric problems.

Reference

1 Susser E, Struening EL, Conover S (1989). Psychiatric problems in homeless men. Lifetime psychosis, substance use, and current distress in new arrivals at New York City shelters. *Archives of General Psychiatry* **46**: 845–50.

① Management of homelessness

Needs are multifaceted and care needs to be integrated with outreach programmes to homeless centres, etc., and systematic evaluation of mental, physical (including dental, health), as well as housing, occupational, and benefit requirements. The Care Programme Approach in the UK facilitates this. Specialist homelessness teams, including psychiatric staff, have been developed and may include community psychiatric nurses, occupational therapists, and social workers. Homelessness can represent the lifestyle of least responsibility, even compared to living in hostels. Many homeless people deny mental illness, avoid mental health services, and are non-compliant with medication treatment.

• Identified physical health problems, including life-threatening
  emergencies such as Wernicke's encephalopathy, should be treated.
• Records of previous assessments should be obtained.
• Local protocols should be followed for the management of violence
  and the presence of weapons. The importance of risk assessment is
  self-evident (see ☐ Chapter 5). Problems with poor communication
  may be encountered and need to be addressed.
• An important decision is whether to admit the patient or to manage
  in a place of safety outside hospital.
• Liaison may need to take place with emergency social services
  to consider emergency housing options.
• Admission to hospital should be driven by health needs and not
  to provide temporary accommodation.
• Always discuss with senior colleagues anyone you are discharging
  without fixed accommodation in which to reside.
• The homeless should be referred to Homeless Persons Units which
  will provide emergency placements in overnight shelters or bed and
  breakfast accommodation. In the UK the current trend is to avoid
  reinforcing homelessness by supporting the homeless (for instance
  with soup kitchens for the homeless on the streets).

☠ Legal framework of management

Psychiatric emergencies relating to substance use, psychotic disorders, and deliberate self-harm are considered in other chapters of this book. In terms of mental health legislation, in England and Wales, admission by the police under Section 136 of the Mental Health Act 1983 may take place. This has a maximum duration of 72 h and allows a patient in a public place to be removed by the police to a 'place of safety' such as a police station or hospital. It is probably better for the individual to be taken to a police station initially and formally assessed by a psychiatrist and social worker there with a view to the need for detention under Section 2 or Section 3 of the Mental Health Act 1983, in preference to an individual being taken by police straight to a psychiatric hospital.

There used to be a tendency for Section 4 of the Act, which allows for emergency admission for assessment by any (one) doctor, to be used in such cases. (This also has a maximum duration of 72 h.) The Mental Health Commissioners recommend that two doctors should be involved in the decision to admit a patient to a hospital under the Act, whenever this is possible, so that Sections 2 and 3 of the Act should be used in preference to Section 4. The Code of Practice states that an applicant cannot seek admission under Section 4 of the Act unless: the criteria for admission for assessment are met; *and* the matter is of urgent necessity; *and* there is not enough time to obtain a second medical recommendation.

📖 Further details relating to mental health legislation are given in Chapter 20 of this book.

Deliberate self-harm and suicide

Deliberate self-harm 116
Risk factors for suicide have been recently
  usefully summarized 118
Assessment of suicidal intent and risk of repetition 119
Management/prognosis/prevention of non-fatal
  deliberate self-harm 119
Association of suicide with psychiatric disorders 120
Association of suicide with physical disorders 121
Association with psychiatric hospitalization 122
Association with general practice consultation 123
National Confidential Enquiry into Suicide and Homicide
  in the UK 124
Association with antidepressant therapy 128
Referral pathways 131
Assessment and management 132
Discharge 135
Emergency assessment of capacity 136

Deliberate self-harm is a common cause of admission to general and psychiatric hospitals. During the period from 1995 to 2007, fewer people have been admitted to hospital and nurses have increasingly had a primary role in assessment and management of such individuals. According to the World Health Organization[1], approximately one million people die by suicide each year[2]. Table 7.1 compares features of completed suicide with deliberate self-harm.

References

1 World Health Organization (1992). The ICD-10 Classification of Mental and Behavioural Disorders. Clinical Descriptions and Diagnostic Guidelines. World Health Organization: Geneva.
2 Vijayakumar L (2006). Suicide and mental disorders—a maze? Indian Journal of Medical Research **124**: 371–4.

☠ Deliberate self-harm

1. Suicide—intended death by action—coroner decides England and Wales 4000 per year (1% of deaths). Total of 8 per 100 000 per year. Self-poisoning—more than hanging and cutting, etc. Been declining generally but increasing among young men. Less in times of war.
2. Non-fatal deliberate self-harm (parasuicide, attempted suicide) Intentional self-poisoning/injury without fatal outcome. England and Wales 120 000 per year. Rose in the 1960s, but declined since. Self-poisoning, mostly using prescribed drugs, accounts for 90%. In 50% of cases alcohol is an additional contributing factor.

Motivation
- Failed suicide attempt in 10%
- Cry for help
- Emotional relief from situation/distress
- Hostility/guilt-inducing to influence others
- Gamble/ordeal.

Repeated self-mutilation
This includes, for example, repetitive wrist cutting. Features include:
- Characterized by mounting tension
- Relieved by cutting, which may be the result of endorphin release.

Table 7.1 Comparison of completed suicide with deliberate self-harm

	Completed suicide	Non-fatal deliberate self-harm
Sex	More males	More females
Age	Late middle age	Late teens/early 20s
Marital status	Widow>Divorced>Single >Married	
Social class	Upper and lower Unemployed and retired	Lower and unemployed
Early childhood	Death of a parent	Broken home
Family history	Depression, suicide, alcoholism	Similar episodes
Physical health	Handicapped/terminal illness	—
Personality	—	Antisocial, borderline, histrionic
Season	Spring	—
Diagnosis	Depression 70% Alcoholism 15% Schizophrenia	'Mental distress' Personality disorder 'Reactive' depression
Precipitants	Guilt Hopelessness	Situational crisis
Setting	Planned Alone Suicide note	Impulsive Others present

Risk factors for suicide have been recently usefully cummarized[1]

Demographic factors

- Male
- Increasing age
- Low socio-economic status
- Unmarried, separated, widowed
- Living alone
- Unemployed.

Background history

- Deliberate self-harm (especially with high suicide intent)
- Childhood adversity (e.g. sexual abuse)
- Family history of suicide
- Family history of mental illness.

Clinical history

- Mental illness diagnosis (e.g. depression, bipolar disorder, schizophrenia)
- Personality disorder diagnosis (e.g. borderline personality disorder)
- Physical illness, especially chronic conditions and/or those associated with pain and functional impairment (e.g. multiple sclerosis, malignancy, pain syndromes)
- Recent contact with psychiatric services
- Recent discharge from psychiatric inpatient facility.

Psychological and psychosocial factors

- Hopelessness
- Impulsiveness
- Low self-esteem
- Life event
- Relationship instability
- Lack of social support.

Current 'context'

- Suicidal ideation
- Suicide plans
- Availability of means
- Lethality of means.

Reference

1 National Mental Health Risk Management Programme (2007). *Best Practice in Managing Risk.* D.O.H.: London, Appendix 2.

Assessment of suicidal intent and risk of repetition

- Never ignore threats. Ask if life is worth living, if suicide ideas and plans are still present
- Ask about plans for suicide for the future—both long- and short-term
- Hopelessness regarding the future increases risk of repetition
- Wanted to die? Regret survival/expected to die
- Previous attempts
- Social isolation and social problems
- Life events, e.g. death of spouse, loss of job, criminal charge
- Psychiatric illness requiring treatment
- Enquire also into other factors associated with completed suicide, e.g. elderly divorced man living alone and alcoholic.

Management/prognosis/prevention of non-fatal deliberate self-harm

- Admit to hospital?
- Compulsory detention?
- 20% repeat and 1% die in next year. 10% eventually complete suicide
- Detect and adequately treat depression, etc.
- Social work and counselling, e.g. Samaritans
- Restrict availability of drugs, e.g. prescribed or in chemists, to avoid impulsive overdoses
- For repeated self-mutilation, coordinate 'team' to minimize gain and set limits, e.g. to admit or not to hospital
- Relaxation techniques. Also applied to repeat self-poisoners, but difficult as patient can have last say
- Dialectical behaviour therapy successful in reducing self-harm in those with borderline personality disorder.

① Association of suicide with psychiatric disorders

In a recent review, Rihmer (2007)[1] stated that: 'More than 90% of suicide victims and attempters have at least one current axis I (mainly untreated) major mental disorder, most frequently major depressive episode (MDE) (56–87%), substance use disorders (26–55%), and schizophrenia (6–13%)... Prospective and retrospective studies [2–5] clearly support the evident clinical observation that if patients with major mood disorder commit or attempt suicide, they do it mostly during their MDE (78–89%) and less frequently in dysphoric mania (11–20%), but very rarely during euphoric mania and euthymia (0–7%), indicating that suicidal behaviour in patients with mood disorder is a 'state-dependent' phenomenon' that is more common in the depressive phase. (The axis I refers to DSM-IV-TR.) Table 7.2 is a hierarchical classification of suicide risk factors and their prognostic utility.

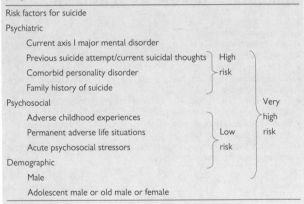

Table 7.2 Hierarchical classification of suicide risk factors and their prognostic utility

Risk factors for suicide

Psychiatric

    Current axis I major mental disorder

    Previous suicide attempt/current suicidal thoughts ⎫

    Comorbid personality disorder   ⎬ High risk

    Family history of suicide   ⎭

Psychosocial   Very high risk

    Adverse childhood experiences   ⎫

    Permanent adverse life situations   ⎬ Low risk

    Acute psychosocial stressors   ⎭

Demographic

    Male

    Adolescent male or old male or female

References

1 Rihmer Z (2007). Suicide risk in mood disorders. *Current Opinion in Psychiatry* **20**: 17–22.
2 Rouillon F, Serrurier D, Miller HD, Gerard 2. MJ (1991). Prophylactic efficacy of maprotiline on unipolar depression relapse. *Journal of Clinical Psychiatry* **52**: 423–31.
3 Isometsa ET, Henrikkson MM, Aro HM, Lonnqvist JK (1994). Suicide in bipolar disorder in Finland. *American Journal of Psychiatry* **151**: 1020–4.
4 Tondo L, Baldessarini RJ, Hennen J *et al.* (1999). Suicide attempts in major affective disorder patients with comorbid substance use disorders. *Journal of Clinical Psychiatry* **60**(Suppl. 2): 63–9.
5 Valtonen H, Suominen K, Mantere O *et al.* (2005). Suicidal ideation and attempts in bipolar I and bipolar II disorders. *Journal of Clinical Psychiatry* **66**: 1456–62.

① Association of suicide with physical disorders

There is evidence that an increased risk of suicide is associated with certain physical disorders, including:

- Cancer[1-3]
- Epilepsy[4,5]
- Multiple sclerosis[1,4,6]
- Migraine with aura[4]
- Stroke[4]
- Traumatic brain injury[4]
- Prostatic disorder, excluding cancer[2]
- Pulmonary disease[2,7]
- Ulcers[2,7]
- AIDS[7]
- Alzheimer's disease[4]
- Huntington's disease[4]
- Parkinson's disease[1].

References

1 Stensman R, Sundqvist-Stensman UB (1988). Physical disease and disability among 416 suicide cases in Sweden. *Scandinavian Journal of Social Medicine* **16**: 149–53.

2 Quan H, Arboleda-Florez J, Fick GH, Stuart HL, Love EJ (2002). Association between physical illness and suicide among the elderly. *Social Psychiatry and Psychiatric Epidemiology* **37**: 190–7.

3 Lefetz C, Reich M (2006). Suicidal crisis in oncology: assessment and care. *Bulletin du Cancer* 93: 709–13.

4 Arciniegas DB, Anderson CA (2002). Suicide in neurologic illness. *Current Treatment Options in Neurology* **4**: 457–68.

5 Jones JE, Hermann BP, Barry JJ, Gilliam FG, Kanner AM, Meador KJ (2003). Rates and risk factors for suicide, suicidal ideation, and suicide attempts in chronic epilepsy. *Epilepsy and Behavior* 4(Suppl. 3): S31–8.

6 Turner AP, Williams RM, Bowen JD, Kivlahan DR, Haselkorn JK (2006). Suicidal ideation in multiple sclerosis. *Archives of Physical Medicine and Rehabilitation* **87**: 1073–8.

7 Goodwin RD, Marusic A, Hoven CW (2003). Suicide attempts in the United States: the role of physical illness. *Social Science and Medicine* **56**: 1783–8.

ⓘ Association with psychiatric hospitalization

Deisenhammer and colleagues[1] have studied all suicides committed in Tyrol, Austria, over a 6-year period in regard to previous psychiatric inpatient treatment. They reported that, of the suicide victims, 16% had been hospitalized at least once. The highest risk for suicide occurred in the period following a recent discharge. Five per cent (representing 28% of those hospitalized) committed suicide within 1 week of discharge, and 8% (representing 48% of those hospitalized) committed suicide within 1 month of discharge. Deisenhammer and colleagues[1] concluded that:

'Whether this hospitalization was driven by the patients or their extra-mural doctors, the increased utilization of psychiatric inpatient treatment reflects an increased need for professional support in mental crises and may be interpreted as a louder cry for help by psychiatric patients...

Periods of increased utilization of psychiatric inpatient treatment constitute high-risk periods preceding a suicidal act and should prompt a particularly profound suicide risk assessment and postdischarge treatment planning.'

While the above study points to the need for suicide risk assessment in those needing psychiatric inpatient treatment, there is evidence that such treatment is itself associated with a reduction in the suicide rate. Qin and colleagues[2] carried out a case-control study based on Danish longitudinal registers of trends in suicide risk associated with hospitalized psychiatric illness. This population-based study included greater than 21 000 suicides which took place in Denmark between 1981 and 1997 (inclusive) and compared them with over 423 000 matched controls. Their results were as follows:

'...the reduction in suicide rate is generally faster among individuals with a history of psychiatric admission than among individuals without such a history. However, this substantial reduction is mainly accounted for by the reduction among patients who had been discharged from psychiatric hospitals for more than 1 year. For patients who had been discharged from hospitals within 1 year, the reduction is similar to that of the general population; while for patients hospitalized for treatment at the time of suicide or the index date, the reduction in suicide is relatively slower. Such trends hold for all diagnostic groups. Further analyses stratified by age indicate that the faster reduction in suicide rate associated with history of hospitalized psychiatric illness is more pronounced among patients aged 36 years and older.'

References

1 Deisenhammer EA, Huber M, Kemmler G, Weiss EM, Hinterhuber H (2007). Psychiatric hospitalizations during the last 12 months before suicide. *General Hospital Psychiatry* **29**: 63–5.
2 Qin P, Nordentoft M, Hoyer EH *et al.* (2006). Trends in suicide risk associated with hospitalized psychiatric illness: a case-control study based on Danish longitudinal registers. *Journal of Clinical Psychiatry* **67**: 1936–41.

⃝ Association with general practice consultation

A recent nested case-controlled study from New Zealand reported that 60% of patients who had died by suicide had had a general practice consultation in the 6 months prior to death[1]. They were more likely than matched control subjects to have: had a previous hospital admission for a psychiatric disorder; a note in their general practice record of depression, suicidal ideation, or self-harm; had a previous hospital admission with self-harm; been prescribed sedatives by their general practice.

Reference

1 Didham R, Dovey S, Reith D (2006). Characteristics of general practitioner consultations prior to suicide: a nested case-control study in New Zealand. *New Zealand Medical Journal* **119**: U2358.

⑦ National Confidential Enquiry into Suicide and Homicide in the UK

Amongst the findings of the National Confidential Enquiry into Suicide and Homicide in the UK, published in 2001, were the following.

Suicides under mental health services

- Approximately one-quarter of suicides had been in contact with mental health services in the year before death; this represents around 1500 cases per year.
- The commonest methods of suicide were hanging and self-poisoning by overdose.
- Mental health teams in England and Wales regarded 22% of the suicides as preventable, with lower figures in Scotland and Northern Ireland, but around three-quarters identified factors that could have reduced risk, mainly improved patient compliance and closer supervision.

Inpatient suicides

- Inpatient suicides, particularly those occurring on the ward, were most likely to be by hanging, most commonly from a curtain rail and using a belt as a ligature.
- Around one-quarter of inpatient suicides died during the first week of the admission.
- Around one-fifth of inpatient suicides were under non-routine observation (constant or intermittent).
- Around one-third of inpatient suicides in England and Wales and Scotland, and almost half of inpatient suicides in Northern Ireland, were on agreed leave at the time of death.

Suicides within 3 months of discharge

- About one-quarter of completed suicides died within 3 months of discharge from inpatient care.
- Postdischarge suicides were at a peak in the first 1–2 weeks following discharge.
- Forty per cent of postdischarge suicides in England and Wales, 35% in Scotland, and 66% in Northern Ireland, occurred before the first follow-up appointment.
- Compared to all community cases, postdischarge suicides were associated with final admissions lasting less than 7 days, readmissions within 3 months of previous discharge and self-discharge.

Non-compliance with treatment

- Around one-fifth of suicides were non-compliant with medication in the month before death.

Missed contact

- Just under one-third of suicides in the community missed their final appointment with services.

Ethnic minorities
- Suicides in ethnic minorities usually had severe mental illness; three-quarters of black Caribbean suicides had a diagnosis of schizophrenia.
- Suicides in ethnic minorities had high rates of recent non-compliance.

Homelessness
- Three per cent of suicides in England and Wales, 2% in Scotland, and 1% in Northern Ireland were homeless or of no fixed abode.
- Seventy-one per cent of suicides among homeless people occurred in inpatients or within 3 months of discharge from inpatient care.

The National Confidential Enquiry into Suicide and Homicide in the UK (2001) included the following recommendations for the prevention of suicide.

New recommendations

Clinical services should place priority for suicide prevention and monitoring on:
- Inpatients under non-routine observations
- Inpatients who are assessed to be at high risk or who are detained and in the first 7 days of admission
- Inpatients who are at high risk and who are sufficiently recovered to allow home leave but whose home circumstances lack support (particularly those who live alone)
- Recently discharged patients who are at high risk or who were recently detained.

Inpatients and postdischarge follow-up
- Inpatient units should remove (or make inaccessible) all likely ligature points.
- Inpatient teams should, in consultation with local service user representatives, develop protocols that allow the removal of potential ligatures from patients who are at high risk.
- Inpatients going on leave should have close community follow-up.
- Patients under non-routine observations should not normally be allowed time off the ward or leave.
- Inpatient services should ensure that there are no gaps, however brief, in one-to-one observation.
- All discharged inpatients who have severe mental illness or a recent (less than 3 months) history of deliberate self-harm should be followed up within 1 week.

Care programme approach (CPA)
- All care plans for enhanced CPA should include explicit plans for responding to non-compliance and missed contact.
- Enhanced CPA should normally apply to patients with schizophrenia, all those with a combination of severe mental illness and self-harm or violence, all homeless patients who have been admitted, and all patients with severe mental illness who are lone parents.

Twelve points to a safer service
- Staff training in the management of risk—both suicide and violence—every 3 years.
- All patients with severe mental illness and a history of self-harm or violence to receive the most intensive level of care.
- Individual care plans to specify action to be taken if patient is non-compliant or fails to attend.
- Prompt access to services for people in crisis and for their families.
- Assertive outreach teams to prevent loss of contact with vulnerable and high-risk patients.
- Atypical antipsychotic medication to be available for all patients with severe mental illness who are non-compliant with 'typical' drugs because of side-effects.
- Strategy for dual diagnosis covering training on the management of substance misuse, joint working with substance misuse services, and staff with specific responsibility to develop the local service.
- Inpatient wards to remove or cover all likely ligature points, including all non-collapsible curtain rails.
- Follow-up within 7 days of discharge from hospital for everyone with severe mental illness or a history of self-harm in the previous 3 months.
- Patients with a history of self-harm in the last 3 months to receive supplies of medication covering no more than 2 weeks.
- Local arrangements for information-sharing with criminal justice agencies.
- Policy ensuring post-incident multidisciplinary case review and information to be given to families of involved patients.

⑦ Association with antidepressant therapy

Prescribing of safer, less toxic, newer psychotropic medications has been held as important in the prevention of suicide, together with restrictions in the sale of analgesics such as salicylates and paracetamol.

It has been suggested that pharmacotherapy with some antidepressants, particularly SSRIs, may be associated with increased risk of suicide, and even of homicide. For example, in their review, Healy and Whitaker[1] concluded that:

> 'These same [randomized controlled trials] … revealed an excess of suicidal acts on active treatments compared with placebo, with an odds ratio of 2.4 (95% confidence interval 1.6–3.7). This excess of suicidal acts also appears in epidemiological studies. The data reviewed here make it difficult to sustain a null hypothesis that SSRIs do not cause problems in some individuals.'

Furthermore, it has been suggested that the increased suicide risk occurs when the SSRI drug dose is being changed, including at the initiation of such pharmacotherapy.

There does indeed appear to be such a risk in those aged 18 years or younger, particularly if unpublished trial results are taken into account[2–4]. On the other hand, at the time of writing there have been several systematic studies and meta-analyses which have failed to detect such a risk in adults[2, 5–10].

In the UK, the Committee on Safety of Medicines (CSM) has issued the following advice relating to the treatment of depressive illness in children, adolescents, and young people (from the *Report of the CSM Expert Working Group on the Safety of Selective Serotonin Reuptake Inhibitor Antidepressants*, December 2004).

Use of SSRIs in children and adolescents

Based on the work of the Group, CSM issued advice on the use of SSRIs in the paediatric population in June, September and December 2003. In summary, that advice was that the balance of risks and benefits for the treatment of depressive illness in under-18s is judged to be unfavourable for paroxetine (Seroxat), venlafaxine (Effexor), sertraline (Lustral), citalopram (Cipramil), escitalopram (Cipralex) and mirtazapine (Zispin). It is not possible to assess the balance of risks and benefits for fluvoxamine (Faverin) due to the absence of paediatric clinical trial data. Only fluoxetine (Prozac) has been shown in clinical trials to be effective in treating depressive illness in children and adolescents, although it is possible that, in common with the other SSRIs, it is associated with a small increased risk of self-harm and suicidal thoughts. Overall, the balance of risks and benefits for fluoxetine in the treatment of depressive illness in under-18s is judged to be favourable.

The safety profiles of the different products in clinical trials in children and adolescents differ across studies. However, an increased rate of a number of events, including insomnia, agitation, weight loss, headache, tremor, loss of appetite, self-harm and suicidal thoughts, occurred in those treated with some of the SSRIs compared with placebo.

Young adults

The increased risk of suicidal behaviour seen in children and adolescents with depressive illness treated with SSRIs raised the question as to whether there was a similar increased risk in young adults. The clinical trial data for each product was reviewed in relation to a possible effect in young adults, and the GPRD (General Practice Research Database) study looked specifically at this age group. From these analyses, the Group concluded that there is no clear evidence of an increased risk of self-harm and suicidal thoughts in young adults of 18 years or over. However, given that individuals mature at different rates and that young adults are at a higher background risk of suicidal behaviour than older adults, as a precautionary measure young adults treated with SSRIs should be closely monitored. The Group also recommended that in further research on the safety and efficacy of SSRIs, young adults should be assessed separately.

Rubino and colleagues[11] have carried out a retrospective UK cohort study of over 200 000 patients comparing the risk of suicide in patients aged 18–89 years during treatment with venlafaxine, citalopram, fluoxetine, and dosulepin. Compared with the SSRIs citalopram and fluoxetine, and the tricyclic antidepressant dosulepin (previously known as dothiepin), venlafaxine use was found to be consistently associated with a higher risk of suicide. However, the authors concluded that, because they had found that venlafaxine was channelled toward patients with more severe and treatment-resistant depression, 'adjustment for measured risk factors could have left residual confounding that could explain some or all of the excess risk associated with venlafaxine.'

References

1 Healy D, Whitaker C (2003). Antidepressants and suicide: risk-benefit conundrums. *Journal of Psychiatry and Neuroscience* **28**: 331–7.

2 Martinez C, Rietbrock S, Wise L et al. (2005). Antidepressant treatment and the risk of fatal and non-fatal self harm in first episode depression: nested case-control study. *British Medical Journal* **330**: 389.

3 Whittington CJ, Kendall T, Fonagy P et al. (2004). Selective serotonin reuptake inhibitors in childhood depression: systematic review of published versus unpublished data. *Lancet* **363**: 1341–5.

4 Hammad TA, Laughren T, Racoosin J (2006). Suicidality in pediatric patients treated with antidepressant drugs. *Archives of General Psychiatry* **63**: 332–9.

5 Fazel S, Grann M, Goodwin GM (2006). Suicide trends in discharged patients with mood disorders: associations with selective serotonin reuptake inhibitors and comorbid substance misuse. *International Journal of Clinical Psychopharmacology* **21**: 111–15.

6 Isacsson G, Holmgren P, Ahlner J (2005). Selective serotonin reuptake inhibitor antidepressants and the risk of suicide: a controlled forensic database study of 14,857 suicides. *Acta Psychiatrica Scandinavica* **111**: 286–90.

7 Gibbons RD, Hur K, Bhaumik DK, Mann JJ (2005). The relationship between antidepressant medication use and rate of suicide. *Archives of General Psychiatry* **62**: 165–72.

8 Khan A, Khan S, Kolts R, Brown WA (2003). Suicide rates in clinical trials of SSRIs, other antidepressants, and placebo: analysis of FDA reports. *American Journal of Psychiatry* **160**: 790–2.

9 Storosum JG, van Zwieten BJ, van den Brink W, Gersons BPR, Broekmans AW (2001). Suicide risk in placebo-controlled studies of major depression. *American Journal of Psychiatry* **158**: 1271–5.

10 Gunnell D, Saperia J, Ashby D (2005). Selective serotonin reuptake inhibitors (SSRIs) and suicide in adults: meta-analysis of drug company data from placebo controlled, randomised controlled trials submitted to the MHRA's safety review. *British Medical Journal* **330**: 385.

11 Rubino A, Roskell N, Tennis P et al. (2007). Risk of suicide during treatment with venlafaxine, citalopram, fluoxetine, and dothiepin: retrospective cohort study. *British Medical Journal* **334**: 242.

ⓘ Referral pathways

Referrals for psychiatric assessment may come from general medical wards, accident and emergency departments, and from the community. Most psychiatric services now have established liaison self-harm teams with psychiatrists and psychiatric nurses with whom accident and emergency departments and general medical wards can liaise closely.

ⓘ Assessment and management

Assessment and management essentially consist of eight steps:
- Establishing fitness for psychosocial assessment
- Immediate management of risk/ensuring safety
- Assessment and documentation of relevant information
- Establishing a psychiatric diagnosis if appropriate
- Risk assessment
- Formulating and documenting a clear management plan in the short medium, and long terms
- Communication of this plan to the patient and appropriate professionals
- Clarifying follow-up options.

Suicide risk assessment needs to be undertaken by all health professionals in contact with patients, and not merely be left to a psychiatrist.

Patients should be asked directly if they have been having suicidal thoughts. There is no evidence that, by so doing, one introduces the idea of suicide into the mind of the patient. On the contrary, at some level the patient may expect this part of their psychopathology to be palpated, and indeed may be relieved to be given an opportunity to ventilate such deeply personal and painful thoughts. Any evidence of suicidal thoughts should be followed by a detailed exploration of the reasons why the patient is considering suicide, and of any method(s) being contemplated, and plans that have been made.

Suicidal thoughts must be taken very seriously indeed. As mentioned above, almost two-thirds of patients who had died by suicide in New Zealand had been found to have had a general practice consultation in the 6 months prior to death[1].

Evidence should be sought for the existence of any of the psychiatric and physical disorders given above which are associated with an increased risk of suicide. Relatives and friends of the patient should be interviewed and information should be obtained about any losses[2], including:
- The break-up of a relationship, including marriage
- Death of a relative or close friend or colleague
- Loss of job
- Financial loss—including gambling debts
- Loss of position or status in society, for instance as the result of being arrested for shoplifting
- Evidence of loneliness and reduced (or no) social contacts.

Scores on Beck's Suicide Intent Scale are useful as a guideline in emergency presentations. The items in this scale include:
- Circumstances related to suicide attempt
  - Isolation
  - Timing
  - Precautions against discovery and/or intervention
  - Acting to gain help during or after the attempt
  - Final acts in anticipation of death
  - Suicide note

- Self-report
  - Patient's statement of lethality
  - Stated intent
  - Premeditation
  - Reaction to the act
- Actual risk
  - Predictable outcome in terms of lethality of patient's act and circumstances known to him
  - Would death have occurred without medical intervention.

The Royal College of Psychiatrists[3] recommends the use of the self-harm assessment form shown in Fig. 7.1, which is adapted from one produced by the Manchester Self-Harm Project at the University of Manchester. This is a useful document that brings together vital aspects of the presentation that can be used specifically to predict risk of future self-harm episodes. It also helps to formulate a clear management plan that can then be communicated between professionals.

Although it is not appropriate to deal in detail with the management of a suicidal patient in this book, the following aspects, taken from Puri et al. (2002)[2] should be taken into account when admitting such a patient to hospital:

> 'If there is a serious risk of suicide the patient should almost always be admitted to hospital, compulsorily if need be. It is important that a good rapport is established between the suicidal patient and the nursing and medical staff, so that the patient can feel free to articulate feelings and thoughts. The patient should be encouraged to be open at all times. Anything that may be used in a suicide attempt, such as sharp objects or a belt (which may be used as a noose) should be removed. Depending on the degree of risk that is judged to exist, the frequency of observation can be varied, for example from every 15 minutes, through an increased level of every 5 minutes, to the highest level of continuous observation. In this case—used when the patient is judged to be at very high risk—a nurse should accompany the patient at all times, including at night (the patient may pretend to be asleep and then get up and attempt suicide by hanging) and in the bathroom (where drowning may be attempted). It may also be useful to nurse such patients in night-clothes (without a pyjama cord, which could be used as a noose) throughout the day, so making it more difficult for them to abscond without being noticed...
>
> Patients with psychomotor retardation are at greater risk of suicide once their symptoms begin to improve. They now have the energy to carry out the act of suicide and they should therefore be observed carefully.'

SELF-HARM ASSESSMENT FORM | ID no.

Patient details	Surname		Date today
	Forename		GP name
	Address		GP address
	Postcode		GP telephone
	Telephone		Hospital
	Date of birth		Hospital number
	Gender: Male ☐ Female ☐		A&E number

Demo-graphic risk factors	Marital status (tick box that applies)
	Single ☐ Separated/divorced ☐ Married/partnered ☐ Widowed ☐
	Ethnic origin (tick most appropriate box)
	White ☐ Black African ☐ Black Caribbean ☐ Chinese ☐ Indian/pakistani/Bangladeshi ☐ Other (please specify) ☐
	Usually living with (tick most appropriate box)
	Street homeless ☐ Alone ☐ Spouse/partner ☐ Parent/sibling ☐ Friends/other relatives ☐ Child(ren) only ☐ Hostel residents/lodgings ☐ Other (please specify) ☐
	Employment (tick most appropriate box)
	Full/part-time ☐ Unemployed ☐ Registered sick ☐ Retired ☐ Homemaker/carer ☐ Student/schoolchild ☐ Other ☐
	If unemployed (tick box that applies)
	Under 26 weeks ☐ Over 26 weeks ☐ Not known ☐

Self-harm details	Method (tick all methods used)
	Self-poisoning, drugs (see below) ☐ Self-poisoning, other ☐ Self-injury (cutting or piercing) ☐ Other (please specify) ☐
	If self-poisoning: tick all drugs that apply and complete boxes as appropriate

Type of drug	*Name*	*No. x dose*	*Type of drug*	*Name*	*No. x dose*
☐ Paracetamol			☐ Opiate		
☐ Other analgesic			☐ Antidepressant		
☐ Antipsychotic			☐ Benzodiazepine		
☐ Other (specify)			☐ Other (specify)		

Alcohol taken within 6 h of harm? Yes ☐ No ☐ How many units? _____

Fig. 7.1 Self-harm assessment form.

References

1 Didham R, Dovey S, Reith D (2006). Characteristics of general practitioner consultations prior to suicide: a nested case-control study in New Zealand. *New Zealand Medical Journal* **119**: U2358.
2 Puri BK, Laking PJ, Treasaden IH (2002). *Textbook of Psychiatry*, 2nd edn. Churchill Livingstone: Edinburgh.
3 Royal College of Psychiatrists (2004b). *Assessment Following Self-harm in Adults.* Council Report CR122. Royal College of Psychiatrists: London.

(7) Discharge

The Royal College of Psychiatrists[1] recommends that the patient information shown in Table 7.3 is obtained before a deliberate self-harm adult
patient is discharged.

Table 7.3 Patient information to be obtained before discharge.
Reproduced with kind permission from the Royal College of Psychiatrists

- Demographic data including ethnicity
- Consciousness level
- Psychiatric history
- Mood
- Presence or absence of thoughts and plans of suicide
- Alcohol and drug misuse
- Previous history of self-harm
- Social situation and events
- Assessment of risk of further self-harm or suicide
- Assessment of capacity to give informed consent
- Decisions taken
- Specific arrangements for any follow-up if not referred on for specialist
  opinion.

Reference

1 Royal College of Psychiatrists (2004b). *Assessment Following Self-harm in Adults*. Council Report
  CR122. Royal College of Psychiatrists: London.

ⓘ Emergency assessment of capacity

If your clinical opinion is that a patient is at high risk of further self-harm, or that they are otherwise in need of further treatment, but they refuse any further medical/psychiatric intervention, then an emergency assessment of capacity is required. This is summarized in the algorithm given in Fig. 7.2.

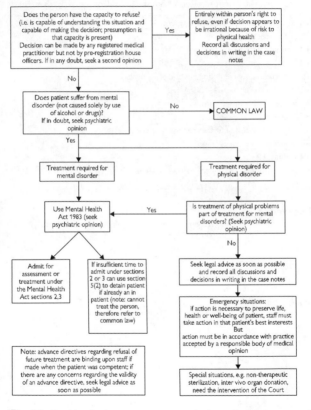

Fig. 7.2 Algorithm for the emergency assessment of capacity. This is an example only, and refers to the Mental Health Act 1983 of England and Wales. Case law is subject to change, and all hospitals and trusts should seek advice from their own legal advisors when developing policy guidance. Reproduced with the kind permission of the Oxford Radcliffe Hospitals NHS trust and the Royal College of Psychiatrics.

Alcohol misuse and dependence

Units of alcohol 138
Levels of consumption 139
Alcohol-related disabilities 140
Alcohol dependence 142
Assessment 144
Acute intoxication 146
Alcohol withdrawal 147

Problems related to alcohol abuse comprise an important part of the accident and emergency department cases in the western world. (Naturally, they are far less common in those countries—predominantly Muslim—in which the drinking of alcoholic beverages is forbidden.) Acute alcohol intoxication-related problems are particularly common on Friday and Saturday evenings/nights, when many, mainly young, people, may become drunk. Chronic alcohol consumption is associated with an increased risk of death from accidents, as well as from cardiac disease, strokes, and cancer.

The total quantity of alcohol per capita a nation drinks is directly related to its relative cost and availability, and is proportional to the prevalence of alcoholism, and alcohol-associated mortality rates.

Excess alcohol consumption (not merely alcohol dependency) is associated with[1]:
• One-third of road traffic fatalities
• A quarter of fatal work accidents
• 30% of drownings
• One-half of deaths from burns.

Alcohol is also involved in[1]:
• A quarter to a third of suicides
• 50–70% of homicides
• Around 60% of assault victims.

Reference

1 Wyatt JP, Illingworth RN, Graham CA, Clancy MJ, Robertson CE (2006). *Oxford Handbook of Emergency Medicine*, 3rd edn. Oxford University Press: Oxford.

Units of alcohol

Between 8 and 10 g of ethanol is contained in a unit of alcohol, which is found in:
• One standard measure of spirits
• A standard glass of sherry or fortified wine
• A standard glass of table wine
• Half a pint of beer or lager of standard (3–3.5% by volume) strength.

One bottle of spirits contains 30 units of alcohol.

Levels of consumption

The Royal College of Physicians' definitions of levels of alcohol consumption are shown in Fig. 8.1.

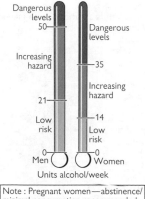

Note : Pregnant women—abstinence/
minimal consumption recommended

Fig. 8.1 Levels of alcohol consumption. Reproduced from Puri BK, Laking PJ, Treasaden IH (2002). *Textbook of Psychiatry*, 2nd edn, by kind permission of Churchill Livingstone, Edinburgh.

⚠ Alcohol-related disabilities

Excess alcohol consumption is associated with physical, psychiatric, and social morbidity.

Physical morbidity

Excess alcohol consumption is associated with increased mortality rates. Causes of morbidity include[1]:

- Gastrointestinal disorders
  - Nausea and vomiting
  - Gastritis
  - Peptic ulcers
  - Mallory–Weiss tears
  - Oesophageal varices
- Malnutrition
- Hepatic damage
  - Fatty infiltration of the liver
  - Alcoholic hepatitis
  - Cirrhosis
- Acute pancreatitis
- Chronic pancreatitis
- Cardiovascular system changes
  - Hypertension
  - Cardiac arrhythmias
- Haematological complications
  - Iron-deficiency anaemia
  - Macrocytosis
  - Folate deficiency
  - Impaired clotting (vitamin K deficiency and/or reduced platelet functioning)
- Cancer
  - Oropharynx
  - Oesophagus
  - Pancreas
  - Liver
  - Lungs
- Fetal alcohol syndrome
- Accidents and trauma
  - Road accidents
  - Assaults—including head injuries
  - Falls—including head injuries
  - Drowning
  - Burns and death by fire
- Infections, e.g. tuberculosis
- Nerve and muscle disorders
  - Myopathy
  - Peripheral neuropathy
  - Cerebellar degeneration
  - Epilepsy
  - Optic atrophy

- Central pontine myelinolysis
- Marchiafava–Bignami disease (primary degeneration of the corpus callosum)
- Psychosexual disorders in men
  - Erectile dysfunction
  - Delayed ejaculation
  - Loss of libido
  - Reduced size of testes
  - Reduced size of penis
  - Loss of body hair
  - Gynaecomastia
- Psychosexual disorders in women
  - Menstrual cycle abnormalities
  - Loss of breast tissue
  - Vaginal dryness.

Psychiatric morbidity

- Mood changes
  - Excess alcohol consumption may be prompted by anxiety or low mood
  - Chronic alcohol consumption is associated with a higher rate of suicide
- Personality changes
- Blackouts
- Delirium tremens 📖 see Chapter 2
- Withdrawal fits
- Alcoholic hallucinosis
  - Auditory hallucinations occur in clear consciousness
  - Noises or derogatory voices
- Pathological (delusional) jealousy
- Fugue states
- Associated with gambling
- Associated with the use of other psychoactive substances
- Wernicke's (alcoholic) encephalopathy 📖 see Chapter 2
- Amnesic or Korsakov's syndrome.

Social morbidity

- Breakdown of relationships, marriages, and families
- Breakdown of friendships and social isolation
- Poor work performance
  - e.g. from hangovers and loss of punctuality
- Crime
  - Arson
  - Sexual offences
  - Violent crimes
- Accidents and trauma
- Driving offences
- Debt.

Reference

1 Puri BK, Laking PJ, Treasaden IH (2002). *Textbook of Psychiatry*, 2nd edn. Churchill Livingstone: Edinburgh.

ⓘ Alcohol dependence

The features of alcohol dependence[1], following chronic heavy drinking, include:
- Primacy of drinking over other activities—including family and career
- Subjective awareness of a compulsion to drink and difficulty in controlling the amount drunk
- A narrowing of the drinking repertoire
- Increased tolerance to alcohol
- Repeated withdrawal symptoms
  - Within 12 h after the last drink: tremor, insomnia, nausea, increasing sweating, anorexia, and anxiety symptoms
  - 10–60 h after the last drink: generalized withdrawal fits
  - After 72 h: delirium tremens
- Relief or avoidance of withdrawal symptoms by further drinking
- Reinstatement after abstinence.

Note that alcohol withdrawal may be the cause of fits in medical and surgical wards (for instance postoperatively).

Reference

1 Edwards G, Gross MM (1976). Alcohol dependence: provisional description of a clinical syndrome. British Medical Journal **1**: 1058–61.

Assessment

History

Look for evidence of the above alcohol-related disabilities. In the alcohol history, take a history of the pattern of drinking, the average number of units of alcohol drunk each week, and any evidence of alcohol dependence, including withdrawal symptoms. The CAGE questionnaire (Table 8.1)[1] should be routinely used to screen for alcohol problems, with a positive answer to two or more of the four questions indicating problem drinking. Note that it is a screening tool and has no place in the assessment of someone with a recognized drinking problem.

Table 8.1 The CAGE questionnaire

C	Have you ever felt you should **C**ut down on your drinking?
A	Have people **A**nnoyed you by criticizing your drinking?
G	Have you ever felt **G**uilty about your drinking?
E	Have you ever had a drink first thing in the morning (an **E**ye-opener) to steady your nerves or get rid of a hangover?

Other routine screening instruments include:
- Fast Alcohol Screening Test (FAST)[2]
- Alcohol Use Disorders Identification Test (AUDIT)[3]
- Severity of Alcohol Dependence Questionnaire (SADQ)[4].

Mental state examination

Look for evidence of psychopathology related to alcohol-related disabilities, such as low mood, confabulation, and delusional (pathological) jealousy.

Physical examination

In the physical examination, particular attention should be paid to the presence of the following (after Puri *et al.*, 2002)[5]:
- Withdrawal symptoms, e.g. tremor, flushing
- Hepatic disease, e.g. liver palms, spider naevi, hepatomegaly
- Accidents or fighting, e.g. haematomas, cuts, broken ribs
- Concomitant illicit drug abuse, e.g. venepuncture marks.

Investigations

It is useful to obtain further information from others, including relatives. For instance, the patient's wife might give a history of alcohol-related domestic violence.

Laboratory investigations which may be helpful include:
- MCV
- GGT
- AST
- Blood alcohol concentration
- Plasma uric acid.

References

1 Mayfield D, McLeod G, Hall P (1974). The CAGE questionnaire: validation of a new alcoholism screening instrument. *American Journal of Psychiatry* **131**: 1121–3.

2 Hodgson RJ, Alwyn T, John B et al., (2002). The Fast Alcohol Screening Test. *Alcohol and Alcoholism* **37**: 61–6.

3 Barbor TF, de la Fuente JR, Saunders J et al., (1992). *AUDIT: The Alcohol Use Disorders Identification Test: Guidelines for Use in Primary Health Care*, 2nd edn. World Health Organization: Geneva.

4 Stockwell T, Hodgson R, Edwards G, Taylor C, Rankin H (1979). The development of a questionnaire to measure severity of alcohol dependence. *British Journal of Addiction to Alcohol and Other Drugs* **74**: 79–87.

5 Puri BK, Laking PJ, Treasaden IH (2002). *Textbook of Psychiatry*, 2nd edn. Churchill Livingstone: Edinburgh.

☣ Acute intoxication

The World Health Organization defines acute intoxication as a transient condition following the administration of a psychoactive substance resulting in disturbances or changes in the patterns of physiological, psychological or behavioural functions and responses. Acute intoxication with alcohol is characterized by slurred speech, incoordination, unsteady gait, nystagmus, and facial flushing, and the differential diagnosis includes head injury, hypoglycaemia, post-ictal states, hepatic encephalopathy, meningitis, encephalitis, and intoxication with other psychoactive substances; a clinical history, mental state examination, physical examination, and appropriate investigations usually allow these possibilities to be excluded (after Wyatt et al., 2006[1]).

The management of patients acutely intoxicated with alcohol presenting to accident and emergency departments, according to their presentation (partly after Wyatt et al., 2006[1]) includes:

- Conscious and ambulant—discharge in the company of a responsible adult is usually appropriate. However, there may be no adults prepared to take responsibility. This can be a very difficult situation for psychiatric trainees. If a patient reports suicide ideation, consideration can be given to detention under the relevant mental health act on grounds of mental illness (depression), as dependency on alcohol or drugs alone is excluded as grounds for detention. In the absence of mental illness relatives may find it difficult to understand why professionals cannot under UK law take action to enforce abstinence. Ultimately, in the absence of mental disorder, a patient is deemed responsible for his actions if he is voluntarily intoxicated, including even if he kills himself.

- Violent—if they appear intoxicated, patients should be examined in a safe environment with access to other staff, panic alarms and, if required, the presence of police (and the results clearly documented) before being escorted from the department by the police (or hospital security); further details on dealing with violent patients are to be found in Chapter 4.

- Comatose—a medical emergency. The patient's airway should be protected and vomiting should be anticipated. Exclude hypoglycaemia and other metabolic causes of coma. Exclude head or neck injury and adopt a low threshold for X-ray and/or CT (or MRI) scanning. Close observation is mandatory.

Reference

1 Wyatt JP, Illingworth RN, Graham CA, Clancy MJ, Robertson CE (2006). *Oxford Handbook of Emergency Medicine*, 3rd edn. Oxford University Press: Oxford.

:⚙: Alcohol withdrawal

This may be treated by the substance misuse services, on an outpatient, day-patient or inpatient basis, depending on the severity of the alcohol dependence. Liaison with general medical teams who may need to undertake the treatment of the individual may be required. Alcohol withdrawal is *not* a psychiatric emergency. A good collaborative working relationship between psychiatrists and the general medical team is required.

Delirium tremens and Wernicke's encephalopathy are emergencies; their management is described in Chapter 2.

Other psychoactive substance misuse

Misuse of Drugs Act 1971 *150*
Opioids *152*
Management of opiate withdrawal *154*
Cannabinoids *156*
Sedatives and hypnotics *158*
Cocaine *160*
Amphetamine and related substances *162*
Caffeine *164*
Hallucinogens *166*
Volatile solvents *170*
History-taking relevant to substance abuse *171*
On examination *171*
Referral to specialist substance misuse services *172*
Investigations *172*
Referral to medical services *172*

A drug modifies one or more functions of an organism. Key definitions include:

- Drug abuse—excessive inappropriate non-medical use to the detriment of health and social functioning
- Drug dependence—compulsion to take the drug to experience psychic effects and/or avoid discomfort of its absence
- Psychological dependence—the drug is taken to produce pleasure or relieve distress (habituation)
- Physical dependence (addiction)
  - Physical symptoms if drug withdrawal (withdrawal symptoms)
  - Associated with tolerance, i.e. with time, less response to same dose and/or need for larger dose for same effect.

It is the comorbidity that is difficult to deal with. For example, the presentation and management of patients with schizophrenia, as inpatients or outpatients, can be compounded by substance misuse. For people presenting with psychosis, there may be a need to distinguish whether their psychosis is drug-induced or represents a functional psychosis.

Substance misuse may be caused by self-medication of symptoms of mental illness. It may also precipitate and/or exacerbate mental illness. An overall assessment of the individual is required. A stress personal vulnerability model can assist in formulation of individual cases. Comorbidity needs to be tackled simultaneously. An individual cannot be detained under the Mental Health Act 1983 in England and Wales for dependency on drugs alone, as this is specifically excluded as a cause alone constituting mental disorder under this legislation.

It is important to be aware of legal (e.g. prescription) sources of psychoactive substances, as well as some of the more common colloquial names used for them, and also the common clinical features of their use and the most likely withdrawal symptoms, to be able to help identify a psychoactive substance aetiology for an emergency presentation.

Misuse of Drugs Act 1971

Under this Act, which applies to England and Wales, the severity of penalties for possession of drugs varies according to class:

- Class A (the most serious) includes opioids, methadone, LSD, mescaline, and cocaine
- Class B includes amphetamines
- Class C—cannabis has been downgraded to this class, but this may be reversed.

① Opioids

Sources

Natural opioids include morphine and heroin, while synthetic ones include methadone and oxycodone. Synthetic substances with opioid agonist and antagonist properties include buprenorphine and pentazocine.

Colloquial names

Colloquial names for heroin include:
- Boy
- Brown sugar
- China white
- Chinese
- Crap
- Dust
- Elephant
- Elephant juice
- H
- Hong Kong rocks
- Horse
- Junk
- Rock'n'roll
- Smack
- Speedball—cocaine mixed with heroin.

Colloquial names for morphine include:
- M
- Morf
- Morpho.

Colloquial names for methadone include:
- Doll
- Dollies.

Clinical features

They are taken legally for use as analgesics and antitussives. Opioids also cause euphoria, with intravenous heroin use being associated with a 'rush' or 'high' which is intense and short-lived. Other effects include:
- Nausea and vomiting
- Constipation
- Drowsiness
- Anorexia
- Reduced libido
- In large doses—hypotension and respiratory depression.

Chronic opioid dependence is associated with:
- Small pinpoint pupils
- Venepuncture marks
- Malaise
- Tremor
- Constipation
- Erectile dysfunction.

Withdrawal symptoms

Opioid withdrawal symptoms, also known as 'cold turkey', include:

- Intense craving for the drug
- Nausea and vomiting
- Lacrimation
- Rhinorrhoea
- Myalgia
- Joint pain
- Mydriasis
- Sweating
- Diarrhoea
- Piloerection
- Yawning
- Insomnia
- Poor body temperature control, e.g. pyrexia
- Restlessness
- Cramp-like abdominal pains
- Tachycardia.

Management

In overdose, cardiorespiratory support and naloxone (an opioid antagonist) may be required. Methadone and clonidine can be used in detoxification. Methadone maintenance is also employed to avoid the worst sequelae of dependency when abstinence cannot be obtained. Needle exchange programmes are employed to counter the risk of infections, including hepatitis and HIV.

Management of opiate withdrawal

- Opiate withdrawal is not in general physically dangerous, except in neonates owing to withdrawal seizures. It may, of course, reveal underlying pain or other physical symptoms
- Symptomatic relief with non-opiate medication:
  - Metoclopramide for nausea and vomiting
  - Zopiclone or zolpidem are better for sleep disturbance than benzodiazepines, with their greater abuse potential
  - Mebeverene for constipation
- Lofexidine (centrally acting α2-adrenergic agonist which reduces noradrenaline from locus coeruleus). Monitor pulse and BP
  - Use 400–600 mcg qds over 7–10 days followed by withdrawal over 2–4 days
- Opioid replacement to control withdrawal symptoms
  - Methadone (a non-injectable opioid agonist) 60–120 mg a day
  - Buprenorphine—a sublingual partial opioid agonist tablet safer in overdose but can be injected. 4–16 mg a day
  - Need hospital pink prescription written in words and figures
- Be clear as to goal
  - Short-term withdrawal
  - Abstinence in longer term as outpatient
  - Maintenance treatment for harm reduction.

ⓘ Cannabinoids

Sources

Natural sources of cannabinoids, particularly of delta-9-tetrahydrocanna-binol, include substances derived from the cannabis plant (hemp or *Cannabis sativa*), such as marijuana and hashish. There are also synthetic analogues of tetrahydrocannabinol available.

Colloquial names

Proper and colloquial names for cannabinoids are given in the following list. The descriptions of potencies refer to the proper use of the names; colloquially, the terms are interchangeable.

- Marijuana—from a mild form of cannabis which tends to be cultivated (often illegally) in the western world
- Hashish or hash—the most potent form, made from pure resin
- Charas—a resinous preparation
- Ghanja or ganja—a preparation made from the flowering tops, leaves, and stems of the cannabis plant
- Bhang—a very mild form
- Kef
- Knif
- Dagga
- Dope
- Grass
- H—more commonly used colloquially to refer to heroin
- Happy stick
- Homegrown—a colloquial name for marijuana
- Joint
- Joy stick
- Paki
- Pot
- Shit
- Smoke
- Tea or Thai sticks
- Weed.

Clinical features

Physical symptoms include:
- Conjunctival injection
- Dry mouth
- Pertussis
- Increased appetite
- Tachycardia.

Psychological effects include:
- Euphoria
- Anxiety
- Suspiciousness—which may develop into persecutory delusions
- A feeling that time is passing more slowly
- Impaired judgement

- Social withdrawal
- Depersonalization
- Derealization
- Hallucinations
- Psychological dependence
- Exacerbates and may predispose or precipitate schizophrenia.

Withdrawal symptoms

Cannabinoids do not cause physical dependence and therefore do not give rise to withdrawal symptoms.

Management

Abstinence.

ⓘ Sedatives and hypnotics

Sources

The main groups of sedatives and hypnotics which may give rise to intoxication (similar to that which may occur with alcohol) are benzodiazepines, barbiturates, and chloral hydrate derivatives.

Colloquial names

Colloquial names for barbiturates include:
- Barbs
- Downers
- Blues
- Nembies—especially for pentobarbitone
- Sodies—especially for sodium amylobarbitone.

Temazepam capsules are sometimes colloquially referred to as jellies.

Clinical features

If a benzodiazepine, such as the contents of temazepam capsules or ground-up tablets, is injected intravenously, this can give rise to a transient 'rush'; venous damage is likely to result. While mild intoxication can present in a similar way to alcohol intoxication, features of increasing sedative or hypnotic intoxication include:
- Slurred speech
- Nystagmus
- Incoordination
- Diplopia
- Strabismus
- Unsteady gait
- Impaired attention
- Impaired memory
- Impaired judgement
- Impaired social and/or occupational functioning
- Hypotonia
- Moderate mydriasis
- Disinhibition—leading to an increase in aggressive, hostile or sexual impulses
- Labile mood.

Chronic use may lead to the development of an amnestic (amnesic) disorder.

Withdrawal symptoms

These may take up to 3 weeks to occur (following last drug use) and include:
- Nausea and vomiting
- Malaise
- Weakness
- Autonomic hyperactivity—including sweating and tachycardia
- Anxiety or irritability
- Orthostatic hypotension
- Coarse tremor of the hands and tongue

- Insomnia
- Grand mal seizures
- Anorexia
- Loss of weight
- Tinnitus.

  Within 1 week of sudden sedative or hypnotic drug cessation, delirium may occur.

Management

Gradual withdrawal, with anticonvulsant cover in the case of barbiturates.

⚠ Cocaine

Sources

The different forms of the alkaloid cocaine are mainly produced from leaves of the coca plant (*Erythroxylum coca*). Clinically cocaine is used as a local anaesthetic. The forms that are (illegally) misused are as follows:

- Coca leaves—which tend to be chewed
- Coca paste—usually smoked
- Cocaine hydrochloride—snorted as a white powder or the solution is intravenously injected
- Crack cocaine—the vapours of the heated form are inhaled, or the substance is smoked.

Colloquial names

Colloquial names for cocaine include:

- Snow
- Coke
- Girl
- Lady
- C
- Big C
- Blow
- Candy
- Cake
- Charlie
- Dust
- Dynamite
- Flake
- Gold dust
- Happy dust
- Happy trails
- Paradise
- Smack
- Snort
- Speedball—cocaine with heroin.

Colloquial names for crack cocaine include:

- Freebase
- Rock
- Base
- Crack.

Clinical features

Cocaine, and even more so crack cocaine, causes strong psychological dependence. Intoxication can lead to:

- Mydriasis
- Tachycardia
- Raised blood pressure
- Sweating
- Nausea and vomiting
- Euphoria
- Grandiosity
- Psychomotor agitation
- Impaired judgement
- Impaired social and/or occupational functioning
- Visual hallucinations
- Tactile hallucinations—formication (the 'cocaine bug').
  With high doses, there may be:
- Ideas of reference
- Increased sexual interest
- Delusional disorder.

Withdrawal symptoms

A rebound crash occurs after the transient rush of using intravenous cocaine or crack cocaine, in which there is:
- Irritability
- Anxiety
- Craving for the drug
- Dysphoria.

Ceasing taking cocaine after a period of chronic use can lead to the following withdrawal symptoms:
- Irritability
- Anxiety
- Craving for the drug
- Dysphoria
- Sleep problems—insomnia or hypersomnia
- Paranoid thoughts
- Suicidal thoughts.

Within 24 h of sudden drug cessation, delirium may occur.

Management

Attempts to decrease craving by use of the tricyclic antidepressant desipramine and other drugs have been made.

① **Amphetamine and related substances**

Sources

Amphetamines (amfetamines) such as dexamfetamine (dexamphetamine) sulphate and related psychostimulants such as methylphenidate hydrochloride are used as prescription medicines in the treatment of attention-deficit hyperactivity disorder. Dexamfetamine sulphate is also used in the pharmacotherapy of narcolepsy. While these legal stimulant drugs are meant to be taken orally, those misusing amphetamine and related stimulant drugs illegally may take them orally, intravenously (for a more intense transient rush) or even by nasal inhalation (as in the case of the abuse of methamphetamine).

Colloquial names

Colloquial names for amphetamine and related stimulant drugs include:
- Speed—particularly for methamphetamine
- Whizz
- A
- Bennies
- Clear rocks
- Crank
- Crystal
- Dexies—particularly for dexamfetamine
- Ice
- Love drug
- Love pill
- M
- Pep pill
- Rocks
- Uppers
- Up.

Clinical features

These include:
- Excitement
- Euphoria
- Increased drive
- Reduced sleep
- Tachycardia
- Mydriasis.

Chronic use is associated with behavioural and psychological effects, including:
- Grandiosity
- Psychomotor agitation
- Hypervigilance
- Impaired judgement
- Impaired social functioning
- Impaired occupational functioning

- Illusions
- Hallucinations—tactile, auditory or visual
- A schizophrenia-like acute psychosis.

Withdrawal symptoms

Ceasing taking amphetamines after a period of chronic use can lead to the following withdrawal symptoms:

- Irritability
- Anxiety
- Dysphoria
- Sleep problems—insomnia or hypersomnia
- Fatigue.

Within 24 h of sudden drug cessation, delirium may occur.

Management

In overdose, sedation, acidification of urine, and anticonvulsant medication may be required. Detoxification is by abstinence with self-resolution of symptoms. Antipsychotic medication may be required if psychotic symptoms are prolonged.

⑦ Caffeine

Sources

The intake of caffeine is legal and widespread in most countries, with common sources including:

- Chocolate—a small bar may typically contain around 5 mg caffeine
- Coffee—one cup typically contains 70–150 mg caffeine
- Tea—one cup typically contains 30–100 mg caffeine
- Cola drinks—one glass typically contains 30–50 mg caffeine
- Caffeine tablets—one tablet typically contains 30–100 mg caffeine
- Aids for losing weight
- Remedies for symptomatic relief from the common cold and influenza.

Clinical features

According to DSM-IV-TR, signs of caffeine intoxication (which occurs after the recent consumption of caffeine, usually more than 250 mg) include:

- Restlessness
- Nervousness
- Excitement
- Insomnia
- Flushed face
- Diuresis
- Gastrointestinal disturbance
- Muscle twitching
- Rambling flow of thought and speech
- Tachycardia or cardiac arrhythmia
- Periods of inexhaustibility
- Psychomotor agitation.

Withdrawal symptoms

According to DSM-IV-TR, features of caffeine withdrawal, which occur after sudden cessation, or reduction in, caffeine consumption following chronic use, include:

- Headache
- Fatigue or drowsiness
- Anxiety or depression
- Nausea or vomiting.

There may also be a strong desire for caffeine-containing products.

① Hallucinogens

Sources

Commonly used hallucinogens include:
- Serotonin-related drugs such as lysergic acid diethylamine (LSD), dimethyltryptamine, mescaline, and psilocybin. The last of these is often consumed from 'magic mushrooms'.
- Phencyclidine and related drugs such as ketamine.
- 3,4-methylenedioxymethamphetamine (MDMA).

Colloquial names

Colloquial names for LSD include:
- Acid
- Acid tabs
- Purple haze
- Blotter acid or blotters
- Paper acid
- L
- Lavender
- Dome(s)
- Dots
- Microdots
- Syd, Sid, or Uncle Sidney
- DSL—the letters of LSD in reverse order
- Rips—probably a shortened form of the word trips
- Ghost
- Alice—from *Alice in Wonderland*
- Lucy in the Sky with Diamonds—from the song with the initials LSD from the Beatles' *Sergeant Pepper* album
- Magic tickets
- Sugar cubes
- Timothy Leary ticket
- Trip
- Sunshine acid.

Colloquial names for mescaline include:
- Mesc
- Cactus
- Buttons
- Peyote
- Pixie sticks
- M
- Dusty.

Colloquial names for psilocybin include:
- Magic mushrooms
- Fun Gus—from fungus
- Fun Guys
- Fungus
- Benzies
- Caps
- Fireworks
- Mucks
- Mushies
- Shroom
- Shroomies
- Toads
- Yellow bentines.

Colloquial names for phencyclidine include:
- PCP
- Angel
- Angel dust
- Dust
- Magic dust
- Peace pill
- Cyclone
- Hog
- Ice
- Juicy—particularly when mixed with cannabis
- Love boat
- Sugar
- Wack.

Colloquial names for ketamine include:
- K
- Keezy
- Vitamin K
- Vetamine
- KFC—which also stands for Kentucky Fried Chicken
- Wonky
- Horse (or Cat, etc.) tranquillizer—after the use of ketamine in veterinary practice
- Special K—after the Kellogg's breakfast cereal
- Kitty.

Colloquial names for MDMA include:
- Ecstasy
- XTC—which is pronounced ecstasy
- Adam
- E
- Beans
- Candies
- Doves
- Eccies
- Egg rolls
- Essence
- Ex
- Love bug
- Love drug
- Love potion
- M
- Jack and jills—Cockney rhyming slang
- Sweets
- Tablets
- Vitamin E
- Vitamin X
- Wingers—a term used in Ulster
- Yips or yokes—used in Dublin.

Clinical features

Physical effects of taking hallucinogens include:
- Tachycardia
- Mydriasis
- Palpitations
- Blurred vision
- Tremor
- Sweating.

Psychological effects include:
• In the case of MDMA, loving feelings towards others, including strangers
• Perceptual abnormalities, including the possibility of hallucinations and synaesthesias
• Depersonalization
• Derealization
• Anxiety
• Impaired judgement
• Impaired social functioning
• Impaired occupational functioning
• Depression—this may lead to suicidal thoughts
• Ideas of reference
• Delusional disorder.

Withdrawal symptoms

With the exception of MDMA, the hallucinogens considered in this section do not, in general, lead to dependency. However, posthallucinogen perception disorders, or flashbacks, may occur a long time after ceasing use of hallucinogens and may be very frightening and stressful for patients, and may cause suicidal thoughts.

Management

As there is no dependence, abstinence is all that is required. Supportive measures, including fluid replacement, may be needed in the case of ecstasy (MDMA).

☠ Volatile solvents

Sources

There are many volatile solvents which are abused, including:

- Solvents
- Adhesives
- Petrol
- Paint
- Paint thinners
- Cleaning fluids
- Butane gas
- Marker pen ink
- Correction fluid
- Spray can propellants.

Clinical features

There is a risk of death from the abuse of volatile solvents in a number of ways, including:

- Suffocation—the solvents are often abused by inhalation from a container such as a plastic bag
- Direct toxicity from the solvent
- Inhalation of stomach contents
- Burns.

DSM-IV-TR gives the following examples of clinically significant maladaptive behavioural or psychological changes occurring during or shortly after use or exposure to volatile inhalants:

- Belligerence
- Assaultiveness
- Apathy
- Impaired judgement
- Impaired social or occupational functioning.

According to DSM-IV-TR, signs of inhalant intoxication include:

- Dizziness
- Nystagmus
- Incoordination
- Slurred speech
- Unsteady gait
- Lethargy
- Depressed reflexes
- Psychomotor retardation
- Tremor
- Generalized muscle weakness
- Blurred vision or diplopia
- Stupor or coma
- Euphoria.

Withdrawal symptoms

With prolonged use, psychological dependence may occur. There is currently no clear evidence of a withdrawal syndrome occurring in humans following chronic use of, or exposure to, volatile solvents.

Management

Abstinence.

History-taking relevant to substance abuse

- Every patient should be asked about illicit and over-the-counter drugs or medication, such as benzodiazepines, which they have obtained from others than their doctor.
- Most young patients will have taken some illicit drugs.
- If a patient admits to taking illicit drugs, ask directly about consumption of all other major categories of illicit drugs.
- For each drug taken, ask about how long taken, escalation, current dose, frequency, pattern of use during week, and route.
- Enquire as to why patient is taking drugs. Is it:
  - To raise mood
  - To reduce social anxiety
  - To 'block' out feelings
  - Due to psychological dependence
  - Due to physical dependence
- Enquire about associated 'risky' behaviours:
  - Infections
  - Sharing needles
  - Sex for drugs
  - Unsafe sex
- Enquire about adverse consequences of drug abuse:
  - Physical
  - Family
  - Occupational
  - Law involvement
- Ask individual about:
  - Do they see drug abuse as a problem and do they believe they can stop
  - Periods of abstinence and reasons for it
  - Triggers to relapse
  - Past treatment
  - Is their social network one of drug abusers.

On examination

- Look for injection sites, abscesses, and DVT.

Referral to specialist substance misuse services

- This should be considered if:
  - Evidence of dependence syndrome
  - Polydrug abuse
  - Associated 'risky' behaviour
  - Pregnancy
- Remember, many GPs are willing and competent to manage and prescribe for substance abusers.

① Investigations

In suspected cases of psychoactive substance use, it is helpful to obtain further information from available and appropriate sources (such as relatives, accompanying friends, and teachers). A drug screen should be carried out in suspected cases of substance misuse, and specific laboratory tests are available for many of the substances mentioned in this chapter.

Referral to medical services

This is indicated if:
- HIV
- Hepatitis B
- TB.
  And urgently if:
- Overdose
- Bacterial endocarditis
- Septicaemia.

NB. Remember opioid withdrawal in adults is not physically dangerous, but benzodiazepine and alcohol withdrawal can be.

Emergencies related to psychotropic drug actions

Acute dystonia 174
Clozapine 175
Serotonin syndrome 176
Hyponatraemia and antidepressants 176
Monoamine oxidase inhibitors (MAOIs) 178
Lithium toxicity 181
Paradoxical reactions to benzodiazepines 181

Neuroleptic malignant syndrome has been considered in Chapter 2.

☠ Acute dystonia

Acute dystonia includes oculogyric crises (📖 see Chapter 2), torticollis, and retrocollis, dysarthria, and dysphagia. It usually occurs at the onset of treatment with antipsychotic medication and is assumed to be caused by an acute hypodopaminergic state in the striatum.

Risk factors include being young, male, and receiving high-potency neuroleptics.

The immediate treatment is parenteral antimuscarinic (anticholinergic) medication, e.g. procyclidine 5 mg IV or IM, or benzatropine (benztropine) 2 mg IV, which can be effective in minutes.

Subsequent management may be by reduction in dose or changes in antipsychotic medication and/or oral antimuscarinic (anticholinergic) medication, e.g. procyclidine 5 mg 8-hourly. Larger doses of procyclidine may produce euphoria, dilated pupils, and are associated with an abuse potential. Diazepam may also help but is less specific.

☠ Clozapine

This archetypal atypical antipsychotic medication is used in treatment-resistant schizophrenia and can be associated with the following fatal side-effects:

- Fatal agranulocytosis—1 in 4250
- Fatal myocarditis and cardiomyopathy—up to 1 in 1300
- Fatal pulmonary embolism—1 in 4500.

On the other hand, it is possible that clozapine treatment may reduce mortality rates in schizophrenia owing to a reduced risk of suicide.

☠ Agranulocytosis

Agranulocytosis occurs in approximately 3% of cases. In the UK, all patients are enrolled with the Clozaril Patient Monitoring Service, which supervises regular blood screening. Each time a blood sample is sent to the Clozaril Patient Monitoring Service, results will be telephoned through if urgent. Otherwise, a typed report alone will be posted.

Examples of telephone communications include:

- No sample received
- Sample not suitable for analysis
- Abnormal haematological results, e.g. neutropenia
  - Clozaril Patient Monitoring Service may advise you to repeat the blood count or stop the clozapine immediately ('red light') and also provide advice about further monitoring.

Examples of written reports include:

- Green light: normal
- Amber light: caution
- Red light: stop clozapine immediately. This will be preceded by urgent telephone contact by the Clozaril Patient Monitoring Service. Daily blood samples will be required until the abnormality is resolved. Specialist haematologist advice may be required. Patients should be monitored for symptoms or signs of infection and not routinely given other antipsychotic medication.

☠ Myocarditis and cardiomyopathy

Fatal myocarditis is most common during the first 2 months of treatment. The UK Committee on Safety of Medicines has recommended:

- Physical examination and medical history before starting clozapine
- Specialist examination if cardiac abnormalities or history of heart disease found—clozapine initiated only in absence of severe heart disease and if benefit outweighs risk
- Persistent tachycardia, especially in the first 2 months, should prompt observation for other indicators for myocarditis or cardiomyopathy
- If myocarditis or cardiomyopathy are suspected, clozapine should be stopped and the patient evaluated urgently by a cardiologist
- Discontinue permanently if clozapine-induced myocarditis or cardiomyopathy.

☠ Withdrawal

Sudden withdrawal of clozapine may be associated with the occurrence of rebound psychosis. If clozapine has to be withdrawn suddenly (see above) then the patient should be observed carefully for signs of psychosis. Otherwise, withdrawal should ideally take place gradually over a 1–2-week period.

☼ Serotonin syndrome

This follows the administration of SSRIs and also lithium salts. It is characterized by:
- Confusion
- Pyrexia and shivering
- Sweating
- Hyperreflexia
- Ataxia
- Myoclonus
- Akathisia
- Tremor
- Diarrhoea
- Poor coordination.

Treatment is by the use of cyproheptadine (which is an antihistaminic, antiserotonin, and anticholinergic medication).

Note that SSRIs can increase the central nervous system toxicity associated with lithium and should not be administered within 2 weeks of an MAOI (monoamine oxidase inhibitor).

☼ Hyponatraemia and antidepressants

The Committee on Safety of Medicines has advised that hyponatraemia should be considered in all patients taking antidepressants (particularly SSRIs) who develop drowsiness, confusion or convulsions. It may be caused by inappropriate secretion of antidiuretic hormone.

:☠: Monoamine oxidase inhibitors (MAOIs)

The use of MAOIs[1]

The enzyme monoamine oxidase (MAO), found mainly in the external mitochondrial membrane, acts on central nervous system neurotransmitters such as noradrenaline, serotonin and dopamine. The involvement of MAO in the metabolic degradation of noradrenaline is shown in Fig. 10.1. MAO catalyzes the catabolism of serotonin into 5-hydroxyindoleacetic acid, or 5-HIAA for short.

Monoamine-oxidase inhibitors, conventionally abbreviated to MAOIs, act by inhibiting the metabolic degradation of monoamines by MAO. The differing actions of MAO-A and MAO-B are shown in Fig. 10.2.

Traditional MAOIs are non-selective, inhibiting the actions of both MAO-A and MAO-B (see Fig. 10.3). Since these MAOIs inhibit the peripheral catabolism of pressor amines, and in particular that of dietary tyramine, it is vitally important that patients taking MAOIs avoid foodstuffs that contain tyramine. Eating tyramine-rich food while taking an MAOI can otherwise lead to a potentially fatal hypertensive crisis. Certain drugs, including over-the-counter medicines like cough remedies, should also avoided avoided while taking MAOIs (see below). These restrictions have tended to limit the use of MAOIs in non-inpatients.

Foods which must be avoided while being treated with MAOIs include
- Cheese (*except* cottage cheese and cream cheese)
- Meat extracts
- Yeast extracts
- Fermented soya bean products
- Alcohol (particularly chianti, fortified wines and beer)
- Non-fresh fish
- Non-fresh meat
- Non-fresh poultry
- Offal
- Avocado
- Banana skins
- Broad-bean pods
- Caviar
- Herring (pickled or smoked).

Medicines which must be avoided while taking MAOIs include
- Indirectly-acting sympathomimetic amines, such as:
  - Amphetamine
  - Ephedrine
  - Fenfluramine
  - Phenylpropanolamine
- Cough mixtures containing sympathomimetics
- Nasal decongestants containing sympathomimetics
- L-dopa

- Opioid analgesics, particularly pethidine
- Tricyclic antidepressants (the combination of the MAOI tranylcypromine with the tricyclic antidepressant clomipramine is particularly dangerous).

The *British National Formulary* (54th edn) gives the following advice on the use of MAOIs before and after (and indeed in addition to) other antidepressants.

> '*Other antidepressants* should **not** be started for 2 weeks after treatment with MAOIs has been stopped (3 weeks if starting clomipramine or imipramine). Some psychiatrists use selected tricyclics in conjunction with MAOIs but this is hazardous, indeed potentially lethal, except in experienced hands and there is no evidence that the combination is more effective than when either constituent is used alone. The combination of tranylcypromine with clomipramine is particularly **dangerous**.

> Conversely, an MAOI should not be started until at least 7–14 days after a tricyclic or related antidepressant (3 weeks in the case of clomipramine or imipramine) has been stopped.

> In addition, an MAOI should not be started for at least 2 weeks after a previous MAOI has been stopped (then started at a reduced dose).

Patients being prescribed MAOIs should be given MAOI treatment cards which list precautions to be taken. These should be issued to the patient by either the prescribing doctor of the dispensing pharmacy.

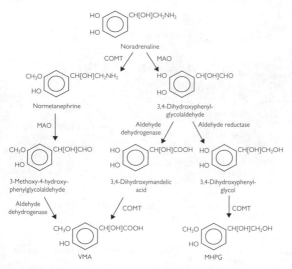

Fig. 10.1 Catabolic pathways for noradrenaline. After Puri *et al.* (2003)[2].

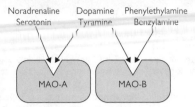

Fig. 10.2 The metabolic degradation of monoamines by MAO-A and MAO-B. After Puri et al. (2002)[2].

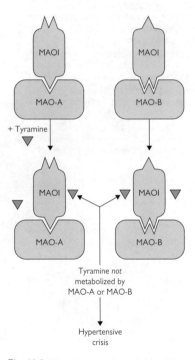

Fig. 10.3 Non-selective and irreversible inhibition of MAO-A and MAO-B by traditional MAOIs. After Puri et al. (2002)[2].

References

1 This section has been reproduced with permission from Puri, BK (2006). *Drugs in Psychiatry*. Oxford: Oxford University Press, pp.168–70.

2 Puri BK, Laking PJ, Treasaden IH (2002). *Textbook of Psychiatry*, 2nd edn. Churchill Livingstone: Edinburgh.

☠ Lithium toxicity

📖 See Chapter 2.

✚ Paradoxical reactions to benzodiazepines

Clinicians have historically been advised in particular of the risk of benzo-diazepines disinhibiting aggression. This was based originally on one item on a scale in one study. While benzodiazepines may disinhibit violence, they can also reduce the risk of violence in those who are particularly tense and anxious.

Acute benzodiazepine withdrawal and acute opioid withdrawal are considered in the previous chapter.

Psychiatric emergencies in accident and emergency departments

Munchausen syndrome (hospital addiction syndrome) *186*
Medically unexplained symptoms *188*

Bruffaerts et al. (2006)[1] studied almost 4000 users of a Belgian university hospital psychiatric emergency room. They found that almost two-thirds were first-time ('incident') users and one-third were recurrent users. Compared with recurrent users, the first-time/incident users were more likely to be:

- Employed
- Referred by a healthcare professional
- Aged over 69 years.

They were also less likely to have:

- A personality disorder
- Used inpatient or outpatient services in the past.

Non-elderly adult attendees presenting with psychiatric emergencies at accident and emergency departments are likely to suffer from one of the following[2]:

- Deliberate self-harm
- Alcohol-related problems
- Other substance abuse
- Delirium and toxic states
- Acute psychoses
- Factitious disorders
- Medically unexplained symptoms.

All but the last two disorders on this list have been discussed earlier in this book. In this chapter, we therefore consider factitious disorders and medically unexplained symptoms.

References

1 Bruffaerts R, Sabbe M, Demyttenaere K (2006). Who visits the psychiatric emergency room for the first time? *Social Psychiatry and Psychiatric Epidemiology* **41**: 580–6.
2 Royal College of Psychiatrists (2004a). *Psychiatric Services to Accident and Emergency Departments.* Council Report CR118. Royal College of Psychiatrists: London.

☠ Munchausen syndrome (hospital addiction syndrome)

Munchausen syndrome is a chronic factitious disorder where physical but also psychological symptoms are voluntarily produced but with an often unconscious motivation. Symptoms are created to assume the sick role, unlike in malingering and also conversion disorder where symptoms are unconsciously produced.

The term Munchausen syndrome was put forward by the psychiatrist Dr Richard Asher in 1951 to refer to those fabricating an illness in order to receive medical attention without secondary gain[1]. Had Asher been less self-effacing, we might now talk of Asher's syndrome (by proxy); one of his daughters, the famous actress Jane Asher, has commented that it was typical of her father not to name the condition after himself. Instead, he named the condition after Karl Friedrich Hieronymus, Baron (Freiherr) von Münchhausen (1720–1797), who achieved fame in his lifetime as a raconteur of tall tales, including those subsequently published in *The Adventures of Baron Munchausen*[2].

In Munchausen syndrome, there is intentional production of feigning of illness to bring about repeated hospital admissions, investigations, and operations. Symptoms simulated suggest severe physical illness and aim to deceive medical staff. Males appear to be affected more than women. The history is plausible but overdramatic. There may be self-inflicted injuries, including simulating symptoms in a bizarre way, e.g. by swallowing needles. Abdominal symptoms are the most common. Pathological lying (*pseudologia fantastica*) is often present. Variations include presenting with psychiatric complaints, including false histories of bereavement, and even psychotic symptoms (factitious psychosis).

When feigning comes to light, such individuals abscond from hospital. They frequently change their name and the hospitals they approach. To fund their wandering they may commit theft and create disturbances. (Note that among those in prison suspected of feigning severe psychotic mental illness, a significant number are found on follow-up to have been genuinely mentally ill. Those feigning mental illness are easily detected. Malingerers will rarely know the characteristic symptoms of schizophrenia and usually present in a histrionic manner. The incongruity between symptoms such as paranoid delusions, and blunted affect, can lead to observers falsely questioning the genuineness of the diagnosis.)

Munchausen syndrome by proxy

This diagnosis was coined by Meadow[3,4]. In Munchausen syndrome by proxy, physical symptoms are intentionally produced in others, for instance, by a mother in her child. The perpetrator frequently has nursing experience. The most often chosen method is poisoning or suffocation. In one-third of cases there is a history of factitious illness in the mother. The father is usually emotionally, if not physically, absent, while the perpetrator appears superficially to be an exemplary mother. One can rarely elicit confessions owing to the offender's shame, low self-esteem, and fear of humiliation.

Management

The Royal College of Psychiatrists[5] have issued the following advice on the management of this disorder in accident and emergency departments.

Management in the A&E department

The management of these patients depends not only on time and resources, but also on the awareness of A&E staff of factitious disorder as a possible diagnosis and on the availability of psychiatric services. When factitious disorder is suspected, the most likely clues are:

- No ascertainable organic cause for the symptoms
- Symptoms and signs suggestive of simulation, e.g. evidence of a ligature around the thigh
- The patient providing no verifiable information, i.e. no address, nearest
- Relative, telephone number or GP.

The patient should be informed that simulated illness is a possibility and asked if a psychiatric assessment would be acceptable. Some patients will decline such an arrangement, and may self-discharge after a non-hostile and supportive confrontation.

The optimum plan of management involves discussion of the patient's history and symptoms with a psychiatrist, followed by joint consultation with the patient. This interview should be supportive rather than adversarial and accusatory, and the patient encouraged to acknowledge that he/she has emotional difficulties for which further help and support may be required.

(Reproduced with kind permission from the Royal College of Psychiatrists.)

References

1 Asher R (1951). Munchausen's syndrome. *Lancet* **1**: 339–41.
2 Puri BK (2006b). Munchausen syndrome by proxy in pregnancy. *International Journal of Clinical Practice* **60**: 1527–29.
3 Meadow R (1982). Munchausen syndrome by proxy. *Archives of Diseases of Children* **57**: 92–8.
4 Meadow R (1989). ABC of child abuse. Munchausen syndrome by proxy. *British Medical Journal* **299**: 248–50.
5 Royal College of Psychiatrists (2004a). *Psychiatric Services to Accident and Emergency Departments.* Council Report CR118. Royal College of Psychiatrists: London.

⚠ Medically unexplained symptoms

The Royal College of Psychiatrists[1] note that patients with medically unexplained symptoms may accumulate rather large folders for their hospital notes, and make the following recommendations for their management.

Management in the A&E department

Management of patients with medically unexplained symptoms in the A&E department depends in part on the doctors' knowledge of the patient's previous medical history. Exploration of the patient's medical history might reveal previous consultation for similar complaints, and enquiries should be made about any other outpatient clinic(s) that the patient may be attending. For example, a subset of female patients with chronic pelvic pain may be attending both gynaecology and gastroenterology outpatient departments.

If the patient is already known to the medical/surgical services, the symptoms are known to be unrelated to organic disease, and there is evidence of psychological distress, e.g. panic attacks, then in certain circumstances it may be appropriate not to perform further medical investigations. The reason for adopting such a conservative, non-interventionist approach is that further tests in such a patient may have iatrogenic potential. For example, the ECG in the patient with non-cardiac chest pain might inadvertently increase that patient's anxiety and lead to further unnecessary consultations (the patient may think 'the doctor wouldn't have done the ECG if he didn't think there was something wrong').

For this reason, it is appropriate for the A&E doctor to attempt to provide a satisfactory alternative explanation for the symptoms in these patients, e.g. hyperventilation or oesophageal reflux in patients with non-cardiac chest pain. Many patients will be reassured by such an explanation, particularly if they feel that they have been listened to and understood by the assessing doctor.

Recommendations

- The management of patients with medically unexplained symptoms depends to a large extent on the A&E doctor's knowledge of the patient's past medical and psychiatric history
- Where available, the use of computerised hospital records would allow A&E staff to identify patients with a previous history of medically unexplained symptoms, especially if they are also attending other outpatient departments in the general hospital
- If the patient's medical complaints are known to be unexplained (or part of a psychiatric illness), then further investigations may be inappropriate.
- The potential to cause iatrogenic harm in these patients should not be underestimated

- These patients should therefore be investigated judiciously, and the indications for use of further investigations carefully considered
- If such patients are also in urgent psychiatric care, then the A&E doctor should communicate with the GP and medical/surgical staff.

(Reproduced with kind permission from the Royal College of Psychiatrists.)

Reference

1 Royal College of Psychiatrists (2004a). *Psychiatric Services to Accident and Emergency Departments*. Council Report CR118. Royal College of Psychiatrists: London.

Psychiatric emergencies in general hospital medical wards

Epidemiology 192
Prevention 192
Common emergencies in psychiatry in general
   hospital wards 192
Acute organic mental disorder/acute confusional
   states/delirium 194
Memory disturbance 196
Mood disorder 197
Psychiatric aspects of neurology 198
Psychiatric aspects of epilepsy 200
Huntington's disease (chorea) 200
Cerebral tumours 200
Parkinsonism 201
Multiple sclerosis 201
Neurosyphilis 201
HIV/AIDS 201
Meningitis, encephalitis, and subarachnoid
   haemorrhages 201
Psychological reactions to neurological symptoms 201
Interaction between psychiatric and physical illness 202
Dissociative and conversion disorders 204
Hypochondriacal disorder (health anxiety disorder) 204
Somatization disorder 206
Medically unexplained symptoms 208
Factors influencing response to physical illness 208
Management 209
Body dysmorphic disorder and other
   associated concepts 210
The uncooperative patient 212
Assessment 212
Problem of patients taking leave against medical advice
   before assessment or treatment is complete 213

Epidemiology

- Psychiatric disorder in general hospital patients is common, perhaps in up to 30% of inpatients.
- However, only a very small proportion, around 1–2%, of general hospital inpatients are referred to psychiatrists.
- Early treatment of a psychiatric disorder can lead to better outcomes, not only for the psychiatric disorder, but also for the medical condition.

ⓘ Prevention

- Adequate screening for psychiatric disorder of patients admitted to general hospital wards at admission highlights those at risk of developing psychiatric emergencies and enables prevention.
- In particular, enquiring about any past psychiatric history is essential.
- Recent life events, such as bereavement, separation or divorce, changes or loss of employment, family illness or financial stresses, increase the vulnerability and/or precipitate psychiatric disorder.
- Particular emphasis in the history and on mental state examination regarding mood and alcohol consumption is also self-evidently important. It is necessary to allow adequate time for such screening to be undertaken, and also for conditions of privacy to exist to facilitate such an assessment.
- Speaking to the individual's relatives, with, whenever possible, the individual's agreement, can provide important independent corroboration and information as to the individual's psychiatric vulnerability.
- The availability of a good psychiatric consultation service which can respond rapidly to referrals or, better still, a liaison psychiatrist integrated into the medical team, can allow appropriate psychiatric intervention that may avert full psychiatric emergencies developing. This service can often provide advice on medicolegal decisions, such as capacity. Such services may also help counter maladaptive staff responses to difficult-to-manage or hostile patients.

☠ Common emergencies in psychiatry in general hospital wards

- Causes of psychiatric emergencies in accident and emergency departments, such as deliberate self-harm or substance misuse, may of course continue following admission to general wards.
- Other causes of psychiatric emergencies include:
  - Acute organic mental disorder/acute confusional states/delirium
  - Memory disturbance
  - Mood disorder.

:⚙: Acute organic mental disorder/acute confusional states/delirium

This has been described in Chapter 2. However, misdiagnosis on general hospital wards is not uncommon. In particular, misdiagnosis as dementia or as functional psychosis such as schizophrenia can lead to inappropriate medication treatment and referral for transfer to a psychiatric hospital when the underlying cause is organic and reversible with appropriate medical treatment of the underlying condition.

Epidemiology

- Up to one in ten of admissions to general medical wards may have acute confusional states, with the frequency rising to up to one-third in those over 65 years.
- Acute confusional states are associated with increased morbidity and mortality rates, and increased length of stay in hospital.
- In reality, acute confusional states are medical rather than psychiatric emergencies.

Clinical presentation

Characteristically there is often:

- An acute onset
- A fluctuating course
- Inattention
- Wandering thoughts
- A fluctuating level of consciousness
- Hallucinations, particularly visual, illusions (misperceptions), and nightmares
- As a guide, consider any individual with visual hallucinations as having an organic mental disorder, usually an acute confusional state but occasionally dementia, until proved otherwise
- Drowsy or agitated or restless
- The clinical picture is usually worse at night
- Short-term memory impairment
- Lability of mood
- Fear and apprehension
- Disturbed or apparently 'strange' behaviour, including inappropriate behaviour towards others on the ward, attempts to leave the ward, disconnecting self from medical equipment such as drips, and aggression.

Table 12.1 shows the clinical features that differentiate acute and chronic mental disorders.

Aetiology

The causes of acute confusional states are organic and theoretically reversible, although sometimes acute confusional states are superimposed on chronic organic mental disorders. Most medical conditions can cause an acute confusional state. The following are more common examples:

- Infection: this can range from a mild urinary tract infection in an elderly person to infection with HIV

ACUTE ORGANIC MENTAL DISORDER **195**

- Metabolic disturbance: causes include hypoxia, electrolyte disturbance, and respiratory, cardiac, renal or hepatic failure
- Endocrine disorders such as diabetes mellitus, including insulin-induced hypoglycaemia which can present with aggression, and Cushing's syndrome
- Vitamin deficiencies: such as thiamine deficiency in those who abuse alcohol and vitamin B_{12} deficiency in pernicious anaemia
- Neurological disorder
  - Head injury
  - Ictal or post-ictal states in epilepsy
  - Space-occupying lesions
  - Raised intracranial pressure
  - Cerebrovascular disease
- Drugs
  - Psychotropic drugs may be used symptomatically in acute confusional states but can exacerbate them
  - Benzodiazepines or barbiturates, for instance used as anti-convulsants, may produce acute confusional states through intoxication or withdrawal
  - Antipsychotic medication
  - Antidepressant medication
  - Cardiac drugs such as digoxin and diuretics
  - Antiparkinsonian drugs such as L-dopa
  - Corticosteroids
  - Opiates for analgesia
  - Illicit substances
- Alcohol withdrawal: delirium tremens may appear within a day or so of admission to hospital due to alcohol withdrawal, and is often characterized by visual hallucinations. If untreated, it has a significant mortality rate, e.g. owing to convulsions
- Postoperative: including from the effects of general anaesthesia.

Management

- Identification and treatment of the underlying cause.
- Attention to nursing and environment. This includes keeping the surroundings well lit and continuously orientating the patient to time and place; being particularly conscious of ensuring that adequate introductions take place of staff; and that explanations of, and reassurance about, procedures are given.
- Drug treatment: sedative medication can clearly aggravate an acute confusional state and may exacerbate underlying medical conditions such as hypoxia through sedation. However, symptomatic antipsy-chotic medication such as haloperidol judiciously used can control otherwise unmanageable disturbed behaviour and aggression.
- Always be aware of the potential for drug interactions, including between prescribed psychotropic drugs and drugs prescribed for underlying medical or surgical conditions, and effects of liver disease on drug metabolism. The appendices on drug interactions in the *British National Formulary* can be helpfully consulted.

Table 12.1 Differential diagnosis of acute and chronic organic mental disorders

Acute confusional state/organic mental disorder/psychosis	Chronic confusional state/senile mental disorder/psychosis
Acute onset Disorientation, bewilderment, anxiety, poor attention	Insidious onset
Clouding of/impaired consciousness, e.g. drowsy	Clear consciousness
Perceptual abnormalities (illusions, hallucinations) Paranoid ideas/delusions If delusions and/or hallucinations termed delirium	Global impairment of cerebral functions, e.g. recent memory, intellectual impairment, and personality deterioration with secondary behaviour abnormalities
Fluctuating course with lucid intervals	Progressive course in dementia Static course in head injury and brain damage
Reversible Causes, e.g. infective metabolic toxic, traumatic degenerative, vascular Alcohol/barbiturate withdrawal	Irreversible

① Memory disturbance

Characteristic causes

- Korsakov's (Korsakoff's) psychosis—a dysmnesic (amnestic) syndrome (memorizing deficit) owing to thiamine deficiency (e.g. in chronic alcoholism), affecting mammillary bodies, the wall of the third ventricle, and the medio-dorsal nucleus of the thalamus. This produces parenchymal loss, proliferation of blood vessels, and petechial haemorrhages. It usually follows on from Wernicke's encephalopathy.
- Poor memory for past events, especially short-term memory, with preservation of remote memory.
- Good immediate recall, e.g. repeating seven numbers forwards and backwards but defective learning after delay or distraction.
- Confabulation
  - Filling in of memory deficit by plausible fabrications
  - False recall in association with failure in memory.
- Acute confusional state/organic psychosis/brain syndrome.
- Dementia—a progressive chronic organic confusional state/psychosis/ brain syndrome, e.g. senile, arteriosclerotic/multi-infarct, presenile.

Differential diagnosis

- Depressive/hysterical pseudodementia
- Schizophrenia with reduced attention and concentration but clear consciousness
- Learning disability, where there is impaired learning rather than poor memory
- Severe mania in bipolar disorder.

ⓘ Mood disorder

- Low mood is common, although often undetected, in a general hospital ward
- Loss of health itself is often experienced as a significant psychological loss, and acute stress reactions and stress related disorders to this and, indeed, hospital life are common. This may lead to either anger or learned helplessness
- Premorbid personality traits may determine an individual's reaction to ill-health
- Adverse psychological reactions may be countered by ensuring patients are adequately informed about their illness and their main worries addressed
- Ill-health and hospitalization can, however, precipitate a depressive mental illness
- It remains important to investigate for organic causes (which cannot all be entirely excluded) of depression and anxiety, including:
  - Prescribed drugs, especially antihypertensives such as beta-blockers, digoxin, and steroids
  - Physical conditions including:
    —hypothyroidism or hyperthyroidism
    —malignancy
    —Parkinson's disease
    —multiple sclerosis
    —brain injury
    —cerebrovascular disease, including stroke.

① Psychiatric aspects of neurology

What are the psychiatric sequelae of head injury?

Psychiatric symptoms and less stable patterns of behaviour are common after severe head injury. Personality/character change and difficult behaviour are among the most tragic consequences. Sometimes they represent not so much a change of personality as exaggeration of previous adverse personality traits. In a family they cause immense stress and depression which may require careful family counselling and support. Psychiatric and behavioural disorder may also sabotage rehabilitation, e.g. of physical sequelae from head injury.

Aetiological factors
- Amount and location of brain damage
- Premorbid personality and past psychiatric disorder
- Family history of psychiatric disorder
- Development of epilepsy
- Poor emotional convalescent environment/home conditions and family support
- Compensation and litigation factors.

Sequelae

Wholly organic in origin
- Impaired/loss of consciousness
- Acute confusional state/delirium
- Retrograde amnesia (before injury, initially lengthy; finally frequently less than 1 minute: not a good prognostic indicator)
- Post-traumatic amnesia (PTA) (anterograde amnesia) is a reliable prognostic indicator
  - The longer the PTA duration, the worse the prognosis
  - In general, if less than 12 h, then full recovery
  - If more than 48 h, probably residual damage
- Cognitive/intellectual impairment (sometimes called dementia—but not progressive)
- Specific deficits, e.g. language difficulties from dominant cerebral hemisphere damage
- Epilepsy can give rise to psychiatric sequelae (described below) associated with epilepsy itself
- Punch-drunk syndrome (e.g. boxers).

Personality change
This is largely organic, but head injury may exacerbate previous personality traits.
- Frontal lobe syndrome: disinhibited, impulsive
- Aggression.

Schizophreniform Psychosis

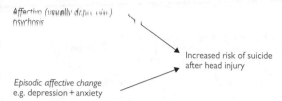

Affective (usually depression)
psychosis

Increased risk of suicide
after head injury

Episodic affective change
e.g. depression + anxiety

NB. Psychosis and suicide more common after temporal lobe damage.

Neuroses
- Commonest psychiatric sequelae
- Depression, anxiety, fatigue, irritability, insomnia; less often obsessional, conversion, and dissociative neurotic disorders
- Increased in 'neurotic' personalities (i.e. head can be more important than injury)
- Less likely if injury in sport or home than, for example, road traffic accident
- More common in minor than in severe head injuries (effort of coping greater after head injury; if injury too severe, patient is unaware of problems and no neurosis results)
- As reaction to physical symptoms: terminology used often overlaps, but includes:
  - Post-concussional or post-traumatic syndrome/neurosis: describes the above symptoms with throbbing headache, dizziness, and poor concentration
  - Merges with compensation neurosis and, rarely, malingering (as does accident neurosis in general). It is more likely if someone else's fault. Symptoms may clear after compensation. Avoid prolonged convalescence.

Overall
Prognosis in head injuries
- Expect improvement to continue for up to 2 years in adults, but longer in children, and may continue for 10 years or more.

① Psychiatric aspects of epilepsy

- Associated with mental retardation (by brain damage, etc)
- In children there may be learning difficulties
- Affects personality development if early onset
  - Particularly temporal lobe epilepsy and if brain-damaged
  - Low sexual drive and sexual deviations
- Neuroses
  - Owing to increased psychosocial stress and stigma
  - Commonest psychiatric disorder
- Pre-ictal
  - Mounting tension, irritability, and gloom.
- Aura
- Ictal
  - Temporal lobe epilepsy leads to mood disturbance, forced thinking, and hallucinations
- Post-ictal
  - Confusional state
  - Automatism, rarely aggression
  - Fugues
- Inter-ictal (between fits)
  - Depression and suicide (risk increased by 5)
  - Chronic paranoid—hallucinatory schizophreniform psychosis (especially dominant temporal lobe epilepsy)
- Increased risk of non-epileptic hysterical conversion pseudoseizures:
  - Variable but often frequent
  - Gradual onset
  - Rigidity and random struggling
  - May be prolonged
  - Usually with others present and at home
  - Emotional precipitant frequent
  - Rarely incontinent or bite tongue or injure self
  - May talk or scream during an attack
  - EEG normal during an attack
  - Serum prolactin not raised after an attack.

① Huntington's disease (chorea)

Autosomal dominant genetic disorder with more than 35 CAG repeats at 4p16.3.
- Psychopathic behaviour with paranoid psychoses and dementia.

① Cerebral tumours

- Fifty per cent present with psychiatric symptoms.

⊕ Parkinsonism

• Depression
  Intellectual impairment.

⊕ Multiple sclerosis

• In 60% there is organic impairment and personality change
• In 50% there is mood change, with early depression and later euphoria
• Risk of misdiagnosis as hysterical.

⊕ Neurosyphilis

GPI (General paralysis of the insane)
• Depression
• Grandiose delusions with psychosis
• Dementia.

⊕ HIV/AIDS

• Depression
• Suicide
• Mania
• Anxiety
• Delirium
• Organic psychosis
• HIV-associated dementia
• Chronic pain leading to substance misuse.

⊕ Meningitis, encephalitis, and subarachnoid haemorrhages

• Brain damage and personality change.

⊕ Psychological reactions to neurological symptoms

• For example, after stroke.

⊘ Interaction between psychiatric and physical illness

Organic mental disorders
- Physical illness has direct effect on brain function
  - Delirium/acute confusional state/organic psychosis, e.g. liver failure
  - Dementia/chronic organic psychosis
  - Postoperative psychosis.

Maladaptive psychological reactions to illness
- Depression, e.g. amputation, mastectomy (due to loss)
- Guilt, e.g. fear of burden on relatives
- Anxiety, e.g. before operation, unpleasant procedure
- Paranoid reaction, e.g. if deaf, blind
- Anger
- Denial
- Preoccupation with illness
- Prolongation of sick role (fewer responsibilities, more attention).

Psychosomatic disease
- Multiple (i.e. biopsychosocial) causes—e.g. life events/stress on physically and emotionally vulnerable leads to changes in nervous, endocrine, and other systems, and disease; for example, bereavement may precipitate a heart attack, or stress may precipitate asthma, eczema, peptic ulcer.

Psychiatric conditions presenting with physical complaints
- Somatic (physical) anxiety symptoms owing to autonomic hyperactivity, e.g. palpitations
- Conversion disorders (via voluntary nervous system)
- Depression leading to facial pain, constipation, hypochondriacal complaints, and delusions, e.g. of cancer, venereal disease
- Hypochondriacal disorder: excessive concern with health and normal sensations.
- Somatization disorder
- Monosymptomatic hypochondriacal delusions, e.g. delusions of infestation or smell; and other psychotic disorders, e.g. schizophrenia
- Munchausen (hospital addiction) syndrome
- Alcoholism leading to liver disease
- Self-neglect.

Physical conditions presenting with physical complaints
- Depressive disorder precipitated by cancer, e.g. of pancreas
- Anxiety in hyperthyroidism
- Post-viral depression, e.g. after hepatitis, glandular fever or influenza.

Medical drugs leading to psychiatric complications
Examples include:

- Antihypertensive drugs leading to depression
- Corticosteroids leading to depression, euphoria
- Antibiotics, e.g. chloramphenicol, streptomycin, cephalosporins, isoniazid, cycloserine, quinolones, may lead to complications such as delirium and psychosis
- Anticancer drugs
- Interferon-α and interferon-β may cause depression and suicide.

Psychiatric drugs leading to medical complications

- Overdoses
- Clozapine, leading to neutropenia.

ⓘ Dissociative and conversion disorders

- In dissociative states, such as amnesia or fugue (unexpected journeying with amnesia), there is partial or complete loss of normal integration between two or more mental processes.
- In conversion disorders there is loss or change in bodily function, usually affecting the voluntary nervous system, such as paralysis or anaesthesia.
- Dissociative and conversion disorders have an unconscious motivation to resolve intrapsychic conflict, and may show the following features:
  - Primary gain (to resolve conflict or reduce anxiety)
  - Secondary gain (e.g. the attention of others)
  - Symptom choice may be symbolic of the conflict and reflect modelling of symptoms that either the individual or others have experienced
  - *La belle indifférence* (patients with la belle indifférence fail to appreciate the significance of their impairments).

Aetiology of conversion disorders

- Predisposing factors
  - Childhood experience of illness
- Precipitating factors
  - Physical illness, e.g. epilepsy
  - Guillain–Barré syndrome
  - Negative life events
  - Relationship conflict
  - Modelling of others' illness
- Perpetuating factors
  - Behavioural responses, e.g. avoidance, disuse, reassurance-seeking
  - Cognitive responses, e.g. fear of worsening, fear of serious disease.

ⓘ Hypochondriacal disorder (health anxiety disorder)

- Disease conviction in spite of medical reassurance
- Intense persistent fear of disease
- Profound preoccupation with body and health status
- Abnormally sensitive to normal physical signs and sensations, and tendency to interpret them as abnormal
- Hypochondriacal symptoms are most frequently secondary to depressive illness.

① Somatization disorder

- A chronic syndrome of multiple physical symptoms not explainable medically
- Increased incidence in first-degree female relatives
- First-degree male relatives have an excess of alcoholism, drug abuse, and antisocial personality disorder
- Unlike hypochondriacal disorder, there is less disease conviction, less fear of disease, and less bodily preoccupation
- Occurs primarily in female, compared to the at-least equal incidence in males of hypochondriacal disorder
- Early onset before 30 years of age, and long course without serious medical illness emerging.

Fig. 12.1 illustrates the spectrum of psychic and somatic symptoms seen in individuals under stress.

Table 12.2 shows the differences in symptoms, motivation, and production of symptoms between somatoform, conversation, dissociative, and factitious disorders.

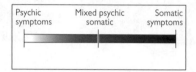

| Psychic symptoms | Mixed psychic somatic | Somatic symptoms |

Fig. 12.1 Spectrum of stress response. Reproduced from Puri BK, Laking PJ, Treasaden IH (2002). *Textbook of Psychiatry*, 2nd edn. Churchill Livingstone: Edinburgh.

Table 12.2 Difference between somatoform, conversation, dissociative and factitious disorders, and malingering

	Physical symptoms	Psychological symptoms	Unconscious motivation	Conscious motivation	Voluntary production of symptoms	Involuntary production of symptoms
Somatoform disorders	+++	−	+	−	−	+
Conversion disorders	++	−	+	−	−	+
Dissociative disorders	−	++	+	−	−	+
Factitious disorders	++	+	+	−	+	−
Malingering	++	+	−	+	+	−

① Medically unexplained symptoms

• Up to one in four non consultations to GPs present with physical symptoms for which no physical cause is found. For new general hospital medical outpatient consultations, this rate is higher, especially in cardiology, gastroenterology, and neurology clinics, where rates may reach 30–50%.

• The current explanatory model of such symptoms is now taken to involve an overlap of the previously considered discrete dissociative, conversion, and somatization models.

• The history given of such symptoms often characteristically includes graphic emotional language, frequent biomedical terms, and attempts to negate explanations from the doctor, including the patient offering his or her own explanations, the citing of additional symptoms when presenting symptoms are explained, and that treatments offered by the doctor on the basis of his or her formulation have been ineffective.

• Always enquire about the effect of such symptoms on daily life, which often appears disproportionate, although the patient may complain that symptoms prevent sleep and thus result in an inability to work.

• Predisposing factors include emotional deprivation in early life, physical illness in early life or in a close family member for whom the patient may also have had to care, life events, and inability to assert one's own needs.

• Unmet emotional needs may lead to the production of physical symptoms which result in and are reinforced by the medical attention and also by collusive carers. There may even be iatrogenic symptoms from inappropriate medical interventions.

② Factors influencing response to physical illness

• Patient
  • Personality (e.g. overanxious, obsessional)
  • Illness behaviour (e.g. at what severity does the patient present)
• Illness
  • Meaning and significance of illness (e.g. cancer)
• Social environment
  • Threat to finances and employment
  • May be welcomed if illness resolves conflict (e.g. marital).

Management

- Physical investigations should only be undertaken and medical treatments only given where clearly medically indicated. To do otherwise, while attempting to reassure a patient that he or she is not seriously medically ill will be counterproductive.
- An attempt to make the patient feel 'understood' should be made, including by acknowledging that the symptoms do feel real for the patient and are not 'all in the mind'.
- An explanation based on a model of stress and psychiatric disorder producing physiological changes and altering perception of normal bodily sensations and/or symptoms, together with the effects of disuse and deconditioning, may be acceptable, understandable, and helpful to such patients.
- The validity of such an explanation may be confirmed to both patient and doctor if previous examples in the patient's life of stress leading to similar physical symptoms are elicited.
- Regular appointments with a GP or psychiatrist can help avoid emergency presentations where the patient's unexplained physical symptoms become a ticket for urgent medical attention. Such regular appointments should attempt to broaden the agenda away from the physical symptoms alone.
- Specific cognitive behavioural treatment can be helpful in minimizing a patient's focus and attention on, and misinterpretation of, physical symptoms and in augmenting healthy perceptions.

ⓘ Body dysmorphic disorder and other associated concepts

- In body dysmorphic disorder (dysmorphophobia) there is a preoccupation with some imagined defect in appearance in a normal-appearing person, which is not of delusional intensity. In these cases there is often comorbid depression or low self-esteem issues. Patients may have a past history of presentation to surgical services.
- In clinical practice most medically unexplained symptoms are caused by undifferentiated somatoform disorder or another primary psychiatric disorder, e.g. somatic anxiety symptoms, facial pain in depression.
- Somatization is the tendency to experience somatic (physical) symptoms unaccounted for by organic causes, to attribute such symptoms to physical illness, and to seek medical help.
- Psychosomatic disorders are physical conditions aggravated or precipitated by psychological factors, e.g. bronchial asthma, peptic ulcer or ulcerative colitis.
- In monosymptomatic hypochondriacal psychosis there are hypochondriacal delusions, such as skin infestation by insects (Eckbom's syndrome) or of an emission of a foul smell.
- Adopting the sick role exempts an individual from normal responsibilities and from being held responsible for the condition.
- Illness behaviour refers to the way symptoms are perceived and acted upon by an individual (see Fig. 12.2) stress disorder.
- Accident neurosis overlaps with post-traumatic. Postconcussional syndrome refers to neurotic symptoms following a head injury.
- In cases of compensation neurosis, symptoms may persist after compensation.
- In malingering, symptoms are consciously produced for an obvious goal, which is lacking in factitious disorders.
- Munchausen's (hospital addiction) syndrome is a factitious disorder where patients repeatedly present at and get admitted to hospitals with feigned symptoms suggestive of serious physical illness.

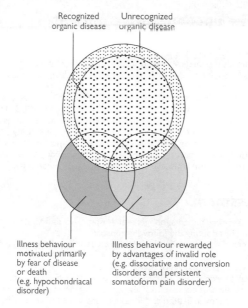

Recognized
organic disease

Unrecognized
organic disease

Illness behaviour
motivated primarily
by fear of disease
or death
(e.g. hypochondriacal
disorder)

Illness behaviour rewarded
by advantages of invalid role
(e.g. dissociative and conversion
disorders and persistent
somatoform pain disorder)

Fig. 12.2 The relationship between organic disease and illness behaviour.
Reproduced from Puri BK, Laking PJ, Treasaden IH (2002). *Textbook of Psychiatry*,
2nd edn. Churchill Livingstone: Edinburgh.

:❂: The uncooperative patient

The cooperation, judgement, and understanding of patients may be adversely affected by the following.
- Fear about the medical condition, its management, and prognosis
- Formal mental disorder such as depression, psychosis, organic mental disorder or learning disability
- Patients who become angry, demanding, or even overtly aggressive may be individuals who otherwise have functioned normally in life but are overwhelmed by what they perceive as intolerable stress
- Alternatively, they may be handicapped by lifelong personality difficulties which may include a lifelong low tolerance to stress with a liability to intemperate outbursts of anger, and, indeed, violence, or a more general antisocial and antiauthoritarian personality.

Assessment

When assessing patients on general hospital wards, diagnosis may be facilitated by adopting the following approach:
- First establish if there is clouding of consciousness, for example by observation of drowsiness and cognitive mental state examination. Be aware that the level of consciousness may vary in acute organic mental disorder/acute confusional state/delirium. If clouding of consciousness is present, this suggests an organic mental disorder, and physical examination and investigations should be directed to finding the cause of this, and the use of sedative drugs to control associated behaviour disorder should be approached with caution
- If there is no clouding of consciousness, does the individual show evidence of positive psychotic symptoms such as delusions (false beliefs) or hallucinations (voices or visions)
  - If yes, then it is likely that the individual suffers from a functional psychosis such as schizophrenia or bipolar affective (mood) disorder
- If there is no evidence of positive psychotic symptoms, mood disorder or neurotic or stress-related disorders should be considered
- Always consider the possibility of intoxication with alcohol or drugs alone or exacerbating other psychiatric disorders.

☠ Problem of patients taking leave against medical advice before assessment or treatment is complete

- If such an individual has a mental disorder of a nature or degree resulting in the individual being at risk to himself, to others, or to his own health, detention under the Mental Health Act 1983 may be appropriate in England and Wales, or under appropriate legislation elsewhere.
- In the absence of detainability under the corresponding Mental Health Act, the individual's capacity to make the decision to leave hospital should be assessed. In the absence of such capacity, the doctor has a duty of care to continue assessment and treatment (the doctrine of necessity), if it is in the individual's best interests.

Considered central to an assessment of capacity are:
- Understanding information relevant to the decision
- Ability to use and weigh up that information as part of the process of making the decision
- Ability to communicate the decision, which can include means other than talking such as sign language or writing
- Capacity should be assessed in relation to a specific decision and time. It is not a global function.

The Mental Capacity Act of 2005, in force since 2007, has introduced designated decision-makers for those who lack capacity for healthcare as well as welfare and financial matters, including Lasting Powers of Attorney and Court-Appointed Deputies. However, the latter will not be able to refuse consent for life-saving treatment. Under this Act formal provision is made for advanced decisions to refuse treatment, including, if expressly stated, 'even if life is at risk'.

Psychiatric emergencies in surgical, radiotherapy, oncology, and terminally ill patients

Psychological consequences of surgery 216
Management of the dying 220
Bereavement 222
Atypical (abnormal) complicated grief 224

① Psychological consequences of surgery

- Between 20 and 40% of patients who have undergone mutilating surgery, including amputation, colonectomy, hysterectomy, and mastectomy, develop mental illness, mainly affective (mood) disorders, which tend to persist for at least a year.
- Factors other than surgery, such as effects of the underlying disease, particularly malignancy, and the unwanted effects of treatment, such as drugs or radiotherapy, may also be relevant.
- Individuals undergoing such surgery may be fearful and uncertain about the prognosis of their condition and of treatments given.
- Feelings of loss and helplessness may develop as a result of such surgery.
- Fear of being shunned by others owing to disfigurement and associated stigma.
- Avoidance of others, leading to social isolation, may follow.
- Feelings of 'why me' are common, and often result in anger and resentment.
- Others experience a sense of failure that it may be too late to achieve ambitions they had for their life, or feelings of guilt for perceived past behaviours, although both can be exacerbated by depression.
- Mastectomy can be associated with feelings of loss of femininity and self-esteem, and result in sexual problems.
- Fear of smelling and rejection after colostomy can also lead to sexual relationship difficulties.
- Cytotoxic drugs and/or radiotherapy as treatments for malignancies can result in fatigue, nausea, vomiting, hair loss, amenorrhoea, and impotence.
- Secondary psychological gain from the sick role can predispose to perpetuation of psychological difficulties.
- While most individuals who have mutilating surgery will suffer some adverse psychological effects, it remains the fact that only a minority develop mental illness.
- Those with a family history or a past history of mood disorder are more likely to develop a mood disorder following such surgery.
- Premorbid personality traits may make others more vulnerable. Perfectionists tend to be more vulnerable, while those who have been able to adjust to severe stresses in the past and accept imperfections in themselves are less at risk.
- Being in a secure stable relationship with another is a good prognostic factor.
- Those who fear rejection are more likely to develop an adverse psychological reaction to such surgery.
- Overt, outward disfigurement is likely to have a greater adverse prognostic effect.

- Uncertainty about prognosis may be more difficult to adjust to than a bad prognosis, although care should be taken not to deny individuals all hope.
- Adjustment will also be more difficult for those whose illness affects their employment, financial situation, and relationships.

Predisposing risk factors to negative psychological consequences of surgery

- Overanxiousness
- Depression
- History in family or acquaintances of adverse outcomes to surgery and underlying conditions, such as cancer
- Lack of a confiding relationship
- Lack of support
- Complications of surgery
- Side-effects of other treatments, e.g. drugs, radiotherapies
- Unable to accept loss of limb, breast, or colostomy, etc.

Routine postoperative screening

- Most individuals with mental illness following mutilating surgery are undiagnosed. The first step in management is therefore routine screening and active enquiry of patients about psychiatric symptoms.
- Routine postoperative screening should include enquires about:
  - Global feeling of wellbeing
  - Mood
  - Sleep
  - Degree of resumption of normal social and occupational activities
  - Relationship with partner
  - Resumption of sexual intercourse
  - Body image revulsion, e.g. loss of breast or limb, colostomy bag
  - Phantom limb sensations
  - Open question as to other fears or problems.
- Staff in general hospital wards spend more time and view more positively patients who display positive feelings. The converse applies to those who openly display negative feelings. Awareness of this dynamic is therefore important.

Management

This should include:

- Giving the opportunity to ventilate feelings.
- Remember individuals may go through the stages of grief (anger, despair, and then acceptance) in response to loss of health, breast, limb, etc.
- The provision of adequate, clear, and accurate information.
- Relief from pain.
- Practical support for problems resulting from surgery such as management of a colostomy or a prosthesis following mastectomy.
- Enquiry about and management of sexual and other potential resulting problems. This can include the use of Masters and Johnson sensate focus techniques.

- Mental illness should be diagnosed and treated in the standard way while being aware that physically ill patients may have a lower tolerance for, and be more likely to develop side effects of, psychotropic medication.
- Antidepressants may be indicated for depression, with the patient advised maximum benefit may be delayed for 4 weeks.
- For anxiety, short-term (2–4 weeks) benzodiazepine medication may be required. Anxiety management techniques can also be employed.
- Body image problems may be helped by cognitive-behavioural techniques, including desensitization to the operative site. Reconstruction surgery can also be considered.

ⓘ Management of the dying

● Awareness in those approaching death of their situation is often much greater than is generally assumed, with perhaps at least three-quarters being fully or partially aware, though many do not discuss their situation with hospital staff or relatives.
● Staff need to be aware of the psychological problems and dynamics already described for those who have had mutilating surgery.
● The risk of affective (mood) disorders is increased in those who are dying.
● Management of the dying requires:
  • Adequate relief from distressing physical symptoms, including pain, as required.
  • Confidence by the patient in those providing care that they will strike the right balance between maintaining life and unnecessary suffering.
  • Symptomatic relief from extreme anguish through psychotropic medication as indicated, e.g. minor tranquillizers or antidepressants.
  • It is important for the patient to maintain close ties with relatives and friends.
  • Do not forget those who will be left behind.
  • Relatives and friends may need to be counselled towards accepting the patient's situation and to deal with their own grief before and after the patient's death.
  • A clinician's judgement and experience are often the best indicators of when, what, and how to tell a particular patient he is dying.
  • There is now an expectation in society that doctors will provide to patients the maximum information available about their condition. Allowing the patient to talk about what they understand about their condition and its prognosis first may reveal that the patient is more informed about their condition and prognosis than is apparent. Immediate replies to direct questions from patients as to prognosis without such enquiry are best avoided.

Breaking bad news to patients or relatives

● This can be a difficult and unpleasant task for doctors and other staff, which can in turn lead to their handling the situation less than satisfactorily.
● Be aware of distancing psychological defences to avoid patient's distress or anger and uncomfortable questions, e.g. 'how long will I live?'
● Such defences include empty bland reassurance, saying how the patient feels is normal in the circumstances or attempts to change subject, e.g. away from condition to how the patient feels otherwise.
● A useful approach is to introduce yourself and your position, and to ask to 'have a word'.
● The discussion should take place in an interview room with adequate privacy.
● It can be helpful to acknowledge initially that either the patient and/or relatives must be worried, and explore their current perception of the situation and how it has affected them.

- Following this, one can explain that the reason for asking them to see you is to provide an update about investigations and management of the illness.
- Explanations should be clear and the patient or relative given ample opportunity to absorb what has been said and to ask any questions they wish.
- Information about treatments and prognosis are usually best undertaken by starting by initially giving any good prognostic points and then explaining the bad side.
- Never give a precise time as to how long a patient may live as this is unpredictable.
- Do not remove hope nor give false hope. Hope, it is said, keeps people alive while despair kills them.
- Before discussing the situation with relatives, first explain your intentions about what you are going to say to the patient unless you consider that the best interest of the patient necessitates that he or she should not be told the full news, at least at this stage.
- Try to discover what the relatives want to know.
- End the interview by again asking if the individuals concerned have further questions.
- Be aware that, because of anxiety, individuals may not absorb or register in memory everything that they have been told the first time round and an offer to meet again is often indicated; let them know how you can be contacted.
- If you are worried about the welfare of a relative who, it is important to remember, is not your patient, suggest they see their general practitioner or otherwise ensure the general practitioner is alerted to the situation.

⑦ Bereavement

Grief is a state that follows loss, e.g. bereavement, separations, etc.

Typical uncomplicated grief/bereavement (normal)

- Stunned phase → Mourning phase → Acceptance phase
                    (Max. 6–10 weeks)   (6 months) and readjustment
- Ruminations about deceased, memories and idealization
- Perceptual disturbances, e.g. hallucinations, illusions, 'presence', misidentifications
- Depression, yearning, agitation, guilt
- Body changes
  - Pale skin
  - 'Choked with grief'
- Increased mortality rates from cancer, 'broken heart' (attack), (myocardial infarction), e.g. widows/widowers have increased mortality rates in the 6 months after bereavement
- Searching behaviour
- Mummification: preserving deceased's possessions
- Hostility to carers of deceased
- Intensity proportional to strength of emotional bond
- Duration inversely proportional to ability to form new relationships
- Worse if loss sudden, accidental or unexpected.

① Atypical (abnormal) complicated grief

Chronic excessively prolonged grief, or more severe, inhibited or delayed or atypical grief. Delayed grief is the commonest presentation.
- Persistent difficulty accepting loss, even denying it
- Marked guilt and self-blame
- Idealization of lost relationship/individual
- Intense hostility, especially to those associated with death, including hospital staff
- Hypochondriacal symptoms mimicking illness of deceased
- Anniversary reactions.

The conditions is more common in:
- Vulnerable personalities
- Those with previous psychiatric difficulties
- Those with an overdependent or ambivalent relationship with deceased
- Multiple life events
- Socially isolated—no confiding relationships.

Other reactions include:
- No response at all/relief in its extreme, 'dancing on grave'
- Psychiatric illness
  - Bipolar affective disorder
  - Depression
  - Schizophrenia
  - Anorexia nervosa
  - Antisocial personality change, alcoholism, gambling
  - Physical illness.

Treatment
In general, normal grief does not require specific treatment, although benzodiazepines can be used to reduce autonomic arousal and sleep disturbance. When abnormal grief or clinical symptoms of depression are present, antidepressants can be considered with supportive counselling.
1. Prevention
   - Society attitudes
   - Caring for the dying. Anticipating and attempting to mitigate future problems of family members
   - Encouraging the dying to express fears and expectations to family, who then feel more supportive
   - Reconciliation of divided families at time of terminal illness.
2. Formal rituals/wakes can help by legitimizing and sharing grief
3. Bereavement counselling/psychotherapy
   - Helping the work of grieving, realization (making real the loss), and disengagement
   - 'Working through'—Listen. Encourage to experience and express feelings (especially after funeral is over), including over painful circumstances of loss and to reactivate unpleasant memories

- Explain symptoms, e.g. illusions, plus supportive psychotherapy. Avoid empty reassurance. Be non-judgemental, e.g. fears over causing death of spouse after a row
- Review relationship and idealization, etc. See regularly, may be for several months
- Aim is to get deceased to right perspective, i.e. acceptance and readjustment without guilt or denial
- Restructure life and fill the gap created.

4. Forced guided mourning (cognitive behaviour therapy) if experience of grief inhibited (conceptualized as avoidance behaviour)
   - Patient made to confront evidence of the death, e.g. tasks of visiting grave regularly, looking at old photos
   - Can be harmful if inadequate family support and significant social problems.
5. Can involve other family members who may share grief
6. Exploit social bridges at turning point of grief
7. Self-help groups (beware risk of perpetuation of grief) e.g. CRUSE (National Widows Organization).
8. Drugs, if indicated, e.g.
   - For 'biological' features of depression (but avoid misdiagnosing grief as a depressive mental illness)
   - For other psychiatric or physical illness precipitated
   - Occasionally for short-term use where severe insomnia and panic (beware risk of drug dependence).

Prognosis

The prognosis depends on the following:
- Vulnerability of previous personality, e.g. ability to form new relationships
- Previous psychiatric difficulties
- Overdependent or ambivalent relationships with deceased
- Multiple life events, e.g. loss of more than one relative, loss of house
- Too much pressure to re-orientate, e.g. re-marry too quickly, pregnancy
- Family/friends/situation may inhibit expression of grief, e.g. mother-in-law inhibits daughter-in-law, 'He's my son.'

Psychiatric emergencies in obstetrics and gynaecology

Perinatal psychiatry 228
Post-partum maternity 'blues' 230
Postnatal puerperal depression 232
Puerperal psychosis 236
Role of psychiatric trainee in initial assessment of
   a puerperal woman 239
Other potentially urgent situations relating to pregnancy
   and childbirth 240
Specialist issues to be considered 244

Perinatal psychiatry

- A relatively new specialty of psychiatry dealing with the management of mental health disorders in the antenatal and postnatal periods.
- Psychiatric illness is the most common cause of indirect maternal death and the largest cause of maternal death overall.

Pregnancy

- *Recurrent miscarriages* and *infertility* may be associated with neurotic or mood disorders, particularly given the importance attached to the fertility of women in society and its importance in a woman's self-identity and self-esteem.
- Women who have become pregnant are less likely to develop psychiatric disorder, commit suicide or be admitted to a psychiatric hospital than at other times. This is in spite of pregnancy being a major life event. Theories as to why this may be so include increasing levels of progesterone during pregnancy, which may be sedative and mildly euphoric, increased tolerance levels in general of mothers, and the sense of wellbeing arising psychodynamically from having something 'good' inside, which may subsequently contrast with the reality of having to look after a child. However, maternal stresses and social problems cannot be discounted as potential foci of intra- and post-partum issues.
- Up to two-thirds of pregnant women have some psychological symptoms, especially in the first and third trimesters, particularly anxiety but also irritability, lability of mood, and depression. Excessive worries may develop about possible deformities in the child, stillbirth, and of pain and splitting open at delivery.
- Up to 10% of women do, however, become clinically depressed, particularly in the first trimester, and the risk is increased in those with a previous history of depression, abortion, unwanted pregnancy, and marital conflict. Counselling, supportive psychotherapy, and, on occasion, marital therapy may be required.
- *Hyperemesis gravidarum* (bad morning sickness) is said to be more common and severe among those who are immature or whose pregnancy is unplanned, or who are denying pregnancy.

Post-partum psychiatric disorders

- The post-partum period is a time of increased psychiatric disorder: in some studies an increase of up to 18 times has been found (Fig. 14.1).

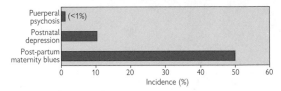

Fig. 14.1 Incidence of puerperal psychiatric disorders. Reproduced with kind permission from Elsevier from Puri et al. (2002). *Textbook of Psychiatry*, 2nd edn.

- Psychiatric disorders termed post-partum are usually taken to include those with an onset up to about 12 weeks following delivery, although other definitions vary from an onset of 6 weeks to up to 1 year post-delivery. Psychoses are similarly referred to as post-partum when onset is from 6 weeks up to 1 year post-delivery. Historically, psychoses whose onset was after 6 weeks were also referred to as *lactational psychoses*.
- Puerperal psychiatric disorders are divided into three main groups, post-partum maternity blues, postnatal depression, and puerperal psychosis, which also have different patterns of onset (Fig. 14.2).
- Clearly, the longer the period from delivery to onset, the less likely there is of a direct relationship between the two.
- In the past, puerperal or lactational psychoses were seen as a specific, unitary psychiatric disorder.
- Nowadays they are seen as a group of psychiatric illnesses, such as depressive disorder or schizophrenia, which can occur at other times. They are not classified separately in ICD-10 or DSM-IV-TR.
- The National Institute of Health and Clinical Excellence (NICE) recommends the use of formal diagnostic categories such as ICD-10 because of the lack of evidence base for the use of the terms postnatal blues, postnatal depression or puerperal psychosis.
- Up until the 19th century and the early part of the 20th century there was a high incidence in the developed world of organic puerperal mental disorders or psychoses, and these are still prevalent in developing countries. These organic disorders were related to infection and loss of blood, but improved maternity services and antibiotics have led to their reduced incidence.

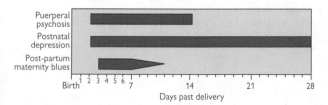

Fig. 14.2 Onset of puerperal psychiatric disorders. Reproduced with kind permission from Elsevier from Puri *et al.* (2002). *Textbook of Psychiatry,* 2nd edn.

① Post-partum maternity 'blues'

- A brief episode of misery and tearfulness that affects at least half of all women after delivery, especially first babies.

Epidemiology

- Following delivery, half to two-thirds of women have a short-lived disturbance of emotions, commencing between the third to fifth days and lasting for 1–2 days, but not beyond 10 days.
- It is more common following the birth of the first child and in those with a history of premenstrual tension.

Clinical features

- These are characterized by episodes of weeping, feelings of depression, anxiety, irritability, feeling separate and distant from the baby, mild hypochondriasis, difficulty in sleeping, and poor concentration.

Aetiology

- It is assumed that post-partum 'blues' have a biochemical and hormonal basis which is associated with the findings of weight loss, reduced thirst, and increased renal sodium secretion.
- It has also been related to normal exhaustion after a climactic delivery following a prolonged pregnancy.
- The onset after 3 days has also been related to the euphoria of delivery being replaced by the reality of having to look after and feed the baby.
- High neuroticism scores on personality assessment have also been found to be more common.

Management

- Once the chronology of presentation is clarified, this requires only reassurance and explanation to the mother and her partner, as the condition is self-limiting within 10 days of delivery.

:Ö: Postnatal puerperal depression

- Any non-psychiatric depressive illness of mild to moderate severity occurring during the first postnatal year.
- Develops later than puerperal psychoses and post-partum maternal 'blues', usually in or after the third week following delivery, peaking in the first 4–6 weeks and overall more common in the first 3 months post-partum than later.
- It affects 70 000 mothers annually in the UK.

Epidemiology

- Occurs in 10–15% of women after childbirth. It is the commonest complication of childbearing.
- This is more likely to occur in those of increased age and lower social class. However, fewer than 1% see a psychiatrist and most receive treatment from their GP or no treatment at all.

Clinical features

- These are similar to those seen in depression at other times, but may be mistaken for normal physiological changes following childbirth, e.g. reduced energy, sleep, and libido.
- Despondency, tearfulness, and irritability are typically seen.
- Fatigue, anxiety, and phobias also frequently occur.
- Mothers develop fears about their ability to cope with their newborn baby and their own and the baby's health.
- Feelings of inadequacy, difficulty in sleeping and concentrating, feeling 'confused', a poor appetite, and decreased libido are also common.
- Guilt feelings can develop over their irritability and their subjective perception of being inadequate mothers.
- Decreased libido, which may be the main symptom, has been related to falling hormone levels.
- The degree of depression itself may be relatively mild or masked, and somatic symptoms may be more prominent. Migraine may be worsened.
- Symptoms are often worse at night. A vicious cycle of worry and insomnia may be set up. The presentation is often one of 'atypical depression', in which there is hypersomnia, hyperphagia, leaden paralysis (heaviness in limbs), and rejection hypersensitivity.
- Mothers painfully contrast their despair with others' observations of how lucky they are to have a newborn child.
- Individuals who develop postnatal depression may be more likely to have high levels of anxiety in the first 3 months of pregnancy, and also during the last trimester, which may then also be associated with admission to hospital for psychosocial reasons, although often ostensibly on clinical grounds, for instance, with proteinuria, oedema, and/or hypertension.
- At interview, the mother's mood should be assessed. Depressive content of thought, including suicidal ideas, if any, need to be elicited, as well as feelings for and attachment to the baby explored.

- Screen for positive psychotic features, such as delusions (false beliefs) or hallucinations (voices), present in the differential diagnosis of puerperal psychosis.
- Fleeting or intrusive thoughts of harming the baby are present in 40% of postnatally depressed women but are rarely acted on.

Investigations

- It is always advisable to visit the family home to assess the home circumstances and to interview the husband or partner.
- The Edinburgh Postnatal Depression Scale (EPDS) is a 10-item self-report screening questionnaire; a score of more than 11 or 12 out of 30 is suggestive of postnatal depression.

Aetiology

- This condition seems predominantly related to the psychological demands of infant care.
- There is little evidence for biological or hormonal factors.
- The risk is, however, doubled by a *previous psychiatric history of depressive disorder* or an *absence of personal social support* from husband, family or friends.
- Some cases may represent mild puerperal psychosis. However, overall there is little evidence for genetic factors. Individuals do not differ from controls in relation to their previous psychiatric history or family history of psychiatric disorder. They also do not differ in their parity. There is an increased history of previous menstrual problems and severe maternal 'blues'.
- Hormonal effects on tryptophan metabolism have been suggested, but not proven, and even adoptive mothers can develop postnatal depression.
- A study of national fish intake in 19 countries found a significant negative correlation between the prevalence of post-partum depression and average fish consumption per person. Countries with a high intake include Japan and Singapore, while countries with a low intake include New Zealand and the United Arab Emirates.
- An association with physical problems during the pregnancy or the postnatal period has been found, especially with caesarian section.
- Lack of a confiding supportive relationship with the partner or other members of the family may predispose towards the development of depression, and this may be associated with social, financial, and marital changes consequent upon the birth of a child.
- Those with postnatal depression are more likely to have had four or more unpleasant significant *stressful life events*, e.g. bereavement or illness, shortly before or during pregnancy. They are also more likely to have had chronic difficulties in their life, e.g. poverty, poor living conditions and physical ill- health, and a poor quality of social support, e.g. from husband or partner, parents, parents-in-law, friends, and a poor social network. These chronic difficulties are present at other times, but the burden of a newborn child may induce helplessness against this background and precipitate postnatal depression.

- It is said that individuals with postnatal depression are in general more neurotic and introverted. Also, postnatal depression may be more common in women with *rigid, obsessional personalities*; those with low self-esteem; those who are *less keen on stereotypical female behaviour* and see little of value in a newborn child after a long pregnancy; those who are *emotionally immature* who may marry too young; and those with *overdependent personalities*, particularly if they are in a mutually over-dependent relationship with their spouse.
- The birth of a child may reactivate a mother's unresolved conflicts such as with her own mother and over her own dependency needs, and bring home to both parents their overdependency on each other. Such a mother may have difficulty caring for a newborn child. There may also be covert hostility to the child.
- Mothers who develop this disorder may be more anxious during pregnancy, for instance if it was the first birth, or if they have a past history of infertility.
- A *disturbed mother–infant relationship* may be causal or caused by postnatal depression. Bonding with a newborn child may be important in preventing postnatal depression. This can be facilitated by the husband or partner being present at delivery, which also decreases the mother's isolation. Research shows that 15 minutes' breastfeeding on delivery is associated with increased eye contact with the child and bonding months later. Postnatal depression is associated with demonstrable disturbance of mother–child interaction, whatever the cause, which then produces a vicious cycle of worsening interactions and further exacerbation of the mother's mental state. Jealousy of the newborn child may lead to *behavioural disturbance in the siblings* and thus additional stress for the mother.
- A mother may develop postnatal depression during one pregnancy and not another because the relationship between her and her husband or partner is changed: each successive pregnancy represents a tightening bond in the marriage. Also, one child may be temperamentally more difficult to manage, e.g. crying more and sleeping less, although this may be due to the circular relationship of the mother's anxiety causing the child to feel insecure.

Management

- It is said that postnatal depression is, for 90% of those suffering from it, a self-limiting condition often lasting less than a month, even without treatment.
- However, *preventative interventions* are important and include education about postnatal depression, good antenatal care with attention to risk factors for postnatal depression, treatment of depression during pregnancy, and support during labour, childbirth, and after the baby is born, e.g. for breastfeeding.
- Supportive psychotherapy and reassurance are of value, as is specific brief psychological therapy, e.g. non-directive counselling or cognitive behaviour therapy.

- It is also helpful to facilitate the involvement of the husband or partner in the newborn's care and to provide practical help to overcome the mother's difficulty in coping
- The involvement of a health visitor can also be of much benefit.
- A group of mothers with similar problems may also be of value.
- If the depression lasts for longer than a month, antidepressants are indicated, and some mothers may respond better to MAOIs than to tricyclic or SSRI antidepressants. However, overall most respond to standard antidepressants. These are secreted in breast milk but are rarely detectable and have not to date been found significantly to affect infants adversely. Nonetheless, clinicians should always consider the potential risks as well as benefits of such treatment for both mother and infant.
- Chronic marital difficulties may require marital therapy.

Prognosis
- Many patients recover spontaneously within 3–6 months without treatment.
- However, one-third to one-half of mothers still have features of postnatal depression at 6 months and 10% at 1 year.
- Overall it is said that 60% are fully recovered within 1 year. Others have residual symptoms and go on to develop a chronic or recurrent mood disorder.
- Research, however, suggests that only 1% see a psychiatrist and that many cases are missed. As a result, such women may continue to suffer from mild depression, with loss of libido often prominent. This sometimes explains why some women state that following pregnancy they are 'never the same again'. A compounding factor in this is that up to one in three women experience painful sexual intercourse in the year after delivery.
- Among primiparae 30% develop depression after a subsequent birth. The rate is increased where the first episode of postnatal depression represents the first ever depressive illness, suggesting that the postpartum period is a specific risk factor.
- Maternal postnatal depression in the absence of adequate fathering or substitute mothering may result in an increased incidence of emotional disturbance in the mother's children, and adverse effects on the next generation of parents and their parenting capacities. Postnatal depression can affect the emotional and cognitive development of the child, especially among boys and in lower social class families. It results in insecure emotional attachments at 18 months and frank behavioural disturbance in boys aged 5 years.
- Given the high rates of undetected and treatable postnatal depression, extra vigilance is necessary from primary care services, i.e. health visitors, midwives, and GPs, to ensure early recognition.

☠ Puerperal psychosis

Epidemiology

- The incidence of puerperal psychosis is at least 1–2 per thousand women but may be as high as 1 in 200 births.
- Results in about 1 in 500 to 1 in 600 women being admitted postnatally to a psychiatric hospital in the UK.
- Excess is owing to affective (mood) psychoses rather than other psychoses such as schizophrenia. It is particularly associated with first pregnancy. One in five has a previous history of bipolar affective (mood) disorder.

Clinical features

- Puerperal psychosis is not a unitary or specific form of psychosis. In the order of frequency of occurrence, it may be:
  - Depressive psychosis
  - Schizophrenia
  - Manic episode
  - Rarely, an organic psychosis, e.g. delirium.
- A few organic psychoses are due to cerebral thrombosis.
- About 70% of puerperal psychoses are affective psychoses and 25% are schizophreniform. However, the nature of the psychosis may only later become clear.
- The grouping of these psychoses together as post-partum psychosis reflects the temporal association of their onset and the striking, acute, florid, unexpected presentation immediately after childbirth in a previously psychiatrically well woman.
- Characteristically there is a *lucid interval*, although this has recently been disputed.
- This is followed by a *prodromal period* of 2–3 days, during which insomnia, irritability, and restlessness may occur, with refusal of food.
- This is then followed by an acute sudden onset of 'confusion' and a rapidly fluctuating clinical picture, with loss of contact with reality, hallucinations, thought disorder, and abnormal behaviour until the exact nature of the psychosis becomes clear.
- Onset is nearly always within the first 2 weeks. The nature and timing are similar to those of postoperative psychosis, possibly suggesting an organic aetiology.
- The clinical presentation, though polymorphic, is usually too overt to miss. Acute onset delusions are usually not systematized.
- The *suicide rate* may be as high as 5% and the risk of *infanticide* as high as 4%. Infanticide in such circumstances is rarely an act of hostility but rather is perceived as one of mercy to prevent suffering of the child.

Aetiology

- Women with a history or family history of bipolar affective disorder or puerperal psychosis are at high risk of developing puerperal psychosis. This suggests that genetic factors are important. The genetic predisposition is, however, less than for such psychoses occurring at other times.

- *Hormonal and biochemical causes* have been suggested as precipitants owing to the sudden decrease in progesterone and luteinizing hormone, the increase in oestrogen and prolactin following delivery, and the resulting effects on tryptophan metabolism and thus on neuro-transmitters, e.g. serotonin (5-HT). However, the evidence for this is not definite.
- Central dopamine receptor sensitivities have been found to be altered.
- There is an increased incidence following first pregnancies. Pre-eclampsia is also more common in first pregnancies.
- *Psychodynamic factors* may be important but have not definitely been established. In general, those who develop psychosis for the first time in the puerperal period have normal personalities and social circumstances and no excess of recent life events. This suggests the importance of biological factors. However, in individual cases the psychosis appears to be precipitated by stillbirth or a child born with a malformation. The stress of the birth may lead to some husbands having a psychotic breakdown and a few women develop an *adoption psychosis* a few days after adoption, which suggests that psychological factors may be more important in some cases.

Management

- Early recognition and treatment is required to avoid possible disastrous consequences for the mother, baby, and family.
- Most mothers require admission to hospital, not only because of the severity and associated behavioural disturbance of their own psychosis, but for the protection of the baby from neglect, mishandling or violence.
- The risk of suicide and infanticide is significant and should always be borne in mind and be assessed.
- Formal Mental Health Act assessment regarding the need for compul-sory detention may be required given the risks and/or absence of insight of the mother.
- Ideally, admission with the child to a mother and baby unit is advisable. This increases bonding between mother and child, and allows supervi-sion and advice to take place. Mothers in general do not wish to be separated from their children and separation in such cases of puerperal psychosis may increase feelings of guilt. However, for some individuals the associated disturbed behaviour is so severe that keeping mother and baby together would not only be impracticable but potentially dangerous. There is some evidence that mothers admitted with their babies do better and stay in hospital for a shorter time than mothers admitted without them. The father should be encouraged to keep in contact with his family unless this is inappropriate for specific reasons. However, the burden of the care of other children may fall heavily on the husband or partner and close family. *Day care* may be an alternative.
- The underlying psychosis should be treated appropriately.
- Treatment options need to be carefully considered and discussed fully with the patient and the family, with appropriate documentation of such discussions.

- Drugs and ECT should be given as appropriate to the symptoms, e.g. antidepressants and/or ECT for psychotic depression, and antipsychotic medication for mania and schizophrenia. A good response to ECT is said to be especially likely in severe puerperal psychotic depression. Antipsychotic medication, however, will be expressed in breast milk; the resulting oversedation of the child may on occasion necessitate the cessation of breastfeeding.
- Supportive psychotherapy is always required, and marital therapy may be required.

Prognosis

- The immediate prognosis is good, with 70% making a full recovery. Those with affective psychosis do better than those with schizophrenia. The risk of a subsequent further episode of psychosis, however, may be up to 50% and up to 20% in any future puerperal periods.
- Those with an affective psychosis are less likely to have further breakdowns when not pregnant, but have an increased chance when pregnant.
- Those with schizophrenia are more likely to have further breakdowns when not pregnant.

⊕ Role of psychiatric trainee in initial assessment of a puerperal woman

The aim is to identify and closely monitor those at risk and detect symptoms characteristic of postnatal depression or post-partum psychosis. The Edinburgh Postnatal Depression Scale (EPDS) is useful in primary care settings. A total score of 12+ is regarded as significant. Always ask about thoughts of self-harm and of harming the baby, especially where the mother remains in contact with the baby, including in mother-and-baby units.

Other potentially urgent situations relating to pregnancy and childbirth

⑦ Couvade syndrome

- This is a dissociative (conversion) disorder in which the prospective father himself develops symptoms characteristic of pregnancy, such as morning sickness, gastrointestinal disturbance, and food craving.
- These symptoms are associated with anxiety and tend to develop either in the first trimester or at the end of pregnancy.
- The syndrome can be seen as understandable anxiety in an overanxious husband. Often there is a strong bond between the couple and overidentification by the male with the future mother.
- There may also be elements of unconscious envy of the woman and her role in childbearing, which may be tinged with hostility. It may also reflect the woman being preoccupied with the pregnancy and less interested in the man.
- Up to 10% of expectant fathers may develop gastrointestinal symptoms at some stage during their wife's pregnancy.
- This syndrome often comes to light incidentally to those caring for the prospective mother. The prospective father needs to be assessed separately from the prospective mother and liaison made with the prospective father's general practitioner.
- Management requires only reassurance, and symptoms usually clear completely following the delivery.

① Use of psychotropic drugs during pregnancy and lactation

Psychotropic drugs may:

- Have a *teratogenic effect* on the developing fetus.
- Result in *withdrawal symptoms* in a newborn baby, if taken by the mother at the end of the pregnancy
- Be present in breast milk fed to the child.

Teratogenic effects

- Severe affective or schizophrenic illness during pregnancy, if untreated, can clearly be a major threat to the wellbeing and sometimes the life of the mother and the unborn child. The issue is one of balancing the risks involved in the illness itself against the risks of continued medication. However, no drug is safe beyond all doubt during early pregnancy.
- A woman may be receiving psychotropic medication during the first trimester before pregnancy is definitely confirmed. Thus a woman's intentions regarding becoming pregnant must always be elicited before prescribing, and prescribing in pregnancy only undertaken when the benefit is thought to be greater than the risk to the fetus.
- However, on present knowledge, if commonly used psychotropic drugs do increase the risk of damage to the fetus, they do not do so to a great extent.

- Typical neuroleptic antipsychotic and older tricyclic antidepressant medications have not been shown to be teratogenic and are probably safe in pregnancy.
- Lithium is regarded as definitely having a teratogenic effect, particularly on the heart, where there is an established risk of Ebstein's anomaly (a cardiac defect with a malformed tricuspid valve).
- There have also been reports of cleft lip and palate in children born to women taking benzodiazepines during pregnancy, although this has been questioned.
- The anticonvulsant phenytoin may produce congenital malformations such as cleft lip/palate, cardiac malformations, and also a fetal hydantoin syndrome of pre-natal growth deficiency, microcephaly, and mental deficiency.
- The effects of excess alcohol in pregnancy, including the 'fetal alcohol syndrome', are well established.

Withdrawal symptoms
- Psychotropic drugs cross the placenta.
- A newborn child may thus show withdrawal symptoms if its mother is dependent on narcotics or alcohol.
- Lithium may result in a baby being born limp or even goiterous.
- Benzodiazepines may result in a '*floppy infant syndrome*' or in other withdrawal symptoms in the newborn, and should thus be avoided.

Effects noted with breastfeeding
- Most psychotropic drugs appear in breast milk.
- However, at standard therapeutic doses, antipsychotic, antidepressant, and anticonvulsant medications have non-significant effects on babies being breastfed milk from their mothers, although the theoretical risk of oversedation should be borne in mind.
- When the mother is taking standard doses of benzodiazepines or lithium, the baby may be adversely affected, and breastfeeding is therefore best avoided.

⑦ Effects on alcohol drinking in pregnancy
Alcohol consumption in pregnancy has been associated with increased rates of stillbirth, neonatal mortality, low birth weight, and problems with attention and distractibility in childhood.

⑦ Fetal alcohol syndrome (FAS)
This is characterized by mental retardation, microcephaly, low birth weight, increased neonatal mortality, cleft palate, ptosis, strabismus, ocular hypertelorism, small nose, long upper lip with narrow vermilion border, scoliosis, pectus excavatum, congenital heart and renal disease, poor growth, and abnormal dermatoglyphia.

Studies suggest it may occur where there is consumption of at least 4–5 units of alcohol daily during pregnancy. The risk with alcoholic mothers is believed to be as high as 20–50%. About 2 in every 1000 live births in the USA have this syndrome.

☼ Opioid dependence and withdrawal in pregnancy

Women who are opioid-dependent and who are either pregnant or who are planning a pregnancy should consider methadone treatment, as the safety of buprenorphine in pregnancy has not been demonstrated.

A newborn child may show withdrawal symptoms if the mother is dependent on opioids.

Beware of the risks of labour analgesia while the mother is on replacement regimens. This is a common scenario where a specialist psychiatric trainee on call may be expected to provide advice.

⑦ Specialist issues to be considered

Mother–infant relationship
- Breastfeeding on delivery is associated with increased eye contact with the child and bonding months later.
- Maternal feelings for a newborn child may normally be delayed for up to 3 weeks, and this may need explaining to a mother and husband to avoid feelings of rejection towards the child.
- For the first 3–4 weeks a mother may feel tired, insecure, and find managing the child unrewarding and hard work. A baby's smile often first elicits maternal feelings.
- By 3 months mothers feel pangs of guilt when they leave their baby.

Stillbirth
- Both mothers and fathers undergo the bereavement process following a stillbirth.
- The psychological effects of stillbirth and the need for counselling have been increasingly recognized.
- Mothers are now encouraged to see and handle stillborn babies, particularly as their imagined perception of the stillborn is usually worse than the reality.
- Fifty per cent of mothers become pregnant again within 1 year, mostly on a planned basis to replace the lost child. Compared with those who become pregnant after 1 year, they show more anxiety during pregnancy, and more depression and anxiety in the year following delivery, perhaps reflecting insufficient grieving of the stillbirth or other vulnerabilities, including of personality.

Oral contraception
- In spite of earlier concerns that oral contraception was associated with, precipitated, or exacerbated severe mental illnesses (such as depression) and reduced libido, more recent research has found only a mild increase in psychiatric symptoms in those with a past psychiatric history, and then only in the first month of oral contraception use.
- Pyridoxine deficiency was found to be associated with depression in a small number on the pill, and thus oral pyridoxine was recommended for administration with oral contraception.

Termination of pregnancy
- Under the Abortion Act 1967 of England and Wales termination is possible:
  - If the continuation of the pregnancy would involve risk to the life of the woman, injury to her physical or mental health or that of existing children in her family greater than if the pregnancy were terminated
  - If there is a substantial risk that, if the child is born, it would suffer from such mental or physical abnormality as to be seriously handicapped.

- In contrast to after the introduction of the Act, psychiatrists are now rarely involved in assessing women requesting termination of pregnancy. Most assessments are now undertaken by GPs and gynaecologists.
- As a general rule, the risk of severe psychiatric disorder following termination of pregnancy is less than for the pregnancy proceeding, i.e. one-fifth of the puerperal psychosis rate. In fact, there is a minority of women who have a history of pregnancy specifically and inevitably resulting in a puerperal psychosis.
- Anxiety and depression are common during unwanted pregnancies but usually resolve within a few weeks of termination.
- There is an increased risk of postnatal depression in women with a past history of termination, unresolved feelings about which may be provoked by giving birth. The more the indications for termination are psychiatric, the greater the risk of post-termination depression. This is also increased in those who are pressurized into having a termination against their wishes.
- Overall, those refused termination have higher rates of regret than those who have had a termination.
- Of those given a termination for depression, over two-thirds subsequently improve.
- Where termination has been refused, among the children born there is evidence to show increased rates of insecurity and delinquency.

Sterilization

- Where the woman is properly assessed and counselled beforehand, sterilization generally results in an improvement in her mental state, wellbeing, marital and sexual relationships, and social adjustment. Overall, there is no increase in psychiatric symptoms, but individuals who are younger, with a small family, and are under pressure to be sterilized are most at risk.

Premenstrual syndrome (late luteal-phase dysphoric disorder)

- Premenstrual syndrome (PMS) consists of emotional, physical, and behavioural symptoms which occur regularly during the second half of each menstrual cycle (i.e. between ovulation and menstruation), subside during menstruation, and are completely absent between menstruation and ovulation.

Epidemiology

- Most women experience some premenstrual symptoms, but of these only 20–40% consider them severe enough to seek medical help.
- For about 6% these symptoms are considered incapacitating.
- The syndrome does not improve with age or parity. Although PMS is found more often in those with other psychiatric disorders, it may be that these sensitize such women to the additional premenstrual changes.

Clinical features
- Over 150 symptoms of PMS have been described.
- Among the most common are *psychological symptoms* such as tension, irritability, depression, fatigue, and poor concentration.
- Physical symptoms include stomach cramps, bloated feeling, backache, breast redness and swelling, swollen fingers and ankles, headache, acne, and weight gain.
- During the premenstrual period there is an increase in parasuicidal acts, suicide, accidents, violent crimes, shoplifting, and poor academic performance.
- Migraine and skin disorders worsen during this period.
- Mothers are also more likely during this period to take their children to see their GP.
- Mental hospital admissions are increased premenstrually, suggesting that PMS exacerbates pre-existing psychiatric disorder.

Investigations and diagnosis
- Diagnosis depends predominantly on confirming the timing of symptoms in relation to menstruation, i.e. symptoms begin in mid-cycle, they increase in number and severity to maximum intensity the day before the onset of menstruation, and this is followed by rapid and complete resolution of symptoms.
- The woman should be advised to keep a diary for at least 2 months of daily ratings of common menstrual cycle symptoms, using a standard symptom record chart to help confirm the diagnosis.

Differential diagnosis
- There is at least a 7-day symptom-free phase after menstruation in PMS. This distinguishes PMS from merely premenstrual exacerbation of other psychiatric disorders, such as depressive disorder or panic disorder, and physical disorders.
- In *dysmenorrhoea* (painful menstruation) the symptoms occur with menstruation, whereas in PMS the symptoms are worst premenstrually.

Aetiology
- The exact cause of PMS is unknown, and different factors may be important in the development of different symptoms.
- Genetic factors have been suggested, as there is an increased incidence in monozygotic compared to dizygotic twins.
- Psychological factors may also have a role. A correlation of PMS with neuroticism has been suggested.
- Physiological factors have also been suggested. Luteal-phase changes in hormones are likely to be important, e.g. a relative deficiency of progesterone, or a rise in oestrogen levels. Alterations in the renin–angiotensin system resulting in excessive aldosterone secretion and fluid retention, pyridoxine deficiency, and alterations in monoamine neurotransmitters with increased MAO activity have also been suggested.

Management

- For many no medical treatment is required, other than information-giving, explanation of the development of symptoms and reassurance including supportive psychotherapy.
- For those more severely affected, target symptoms should be identified and treated, e.g. with *analgesics* if the predominant symptoms are headache or pain, or evening primrose oil, danazol or bromocriptine for cyclical breast pain.
- There is little evidence that progesterones or bromocriptine are more effective than placebo. Progesterone is inactive by mouth and therefore has to be administered in the form of rectal or vaginal suppositories or daily injections. Oral synthetic progesterones, such as dydrogesterone (duphaston), are, however, available. Bromocriptine suppresses prolactin secretion but produces postural hypotension and nausea.
- Diuretics, particularly spironolactone (an aldosterone antagonist), have been used, given the postulated role of fluid retention.
- Pyridoxine, while largely harmless, is of uncertain efficacy.
- Where contraception is also required, the *oral contraceptive pill*, particularly a low-dose combination, may be effective. *Oestrogen* as an implant or transdermal patch has also been used.
- Lithium, antidepressants (particularly the SSRIs), benzodiazepines, and relaxation therapy have also been used to variable and disputed effect.

Menopause

- There is no evidence that severe mental illness is more common in women around the time of the menopause.
- Previous descriptions of a distinct depressive disorder—involutional melancholia—specifically linked to the menopause have not been con-firmed. The clinical picture described then probably merely reflected the characteristic presentation of depressive disorder at that age.
- The menopause may psychologically alter the woman's perception of herself, and often occurs at a time when other major life events are also taking place, e.g. children leaving home, retirement, parents dying.
- Ninety per cent of women do experience hot flushes and excessive sweating for 1–2 years after the cessation of periods, owing to reduced ovarian activity causing vasomotor changes. These respond to oestrogen treatment.
- However, in the year following the menopause, up to one-third of women experience anxiety, irritability, fatigue, and headaches, which is 10% greater than at other times. Such mild affective (mood) disorder during the menopause does not respond to oestrogen therapy any better than placebo.

Hysterectomy
- Although psychiatric referral following a hysterectomy is greater than for other abdominal operations, particularly where no physical pathology was found at operation, research has shown that such individuals had a high level of preoperative psychiatric morbidity, which the operation reduces but to a level still higher than the general population.
- It has been suggested that psychiatric disorder may be associated with menorrhagia (heavy periods), which may necessitate the surgery as a matter of urgency.

① Amenorrhoea
- This can occur following psychological stress and in psychiatric disorders such as depression and anorexia nervosa. Antipsychotic neuroleptic medication results in increased prolactin levels and thus amenorrhoea.

Psychiatric emergencies in children and adolescents

Assessment *250*
Children Act 1989 *251*
Safety issues *251*
Self-harm *252*
Child abuse *254*
Other psychiatric emergencies *256*

Child psychiatric disorder is often a quantitative deviance from the norm with suffering, disturbance, and/or handicap. Child and adolescent psychiatric disorder occurs in 5–20%, being twice as common in boys then girls, higher in urban compared to rural areas, five times higher when brain injury is present, and also increased when physical handicap is present.

Multifactorial aetiology and comorbidity are the rule. A multiaxial classification is used in ICD-10 (version 4), the axes being:
• Clinical syndrome
• Medical condition
• Psychosocial problems
• Special delays in development
• Intellectual level.

Child psychiatric disorder is not necessarily a prerequisite for referral to child and adolescent mental health services, but may reflect disorder elsewhere in the family or environment.

Types of presentation to child and adolescent mental health services include:
• Conduct disorder
• Emotional disorder
• Depression
• Self-harm
• Child protection issues, including non-accidental injury, sexual and emotional abuse, and neglect
• Acute psychiatric crises, including psychoses. These often result in presentation at emergency departments and admission to paediatric wards.

Assessment

An ideal child psychiatric assessment includes a whole family interview, an interview with parents or carers, an interview with the 'identified child', and possible interviews with others, e.g. siblings, social workers, etc.

Areas of assessment include:
1. History of presenting complaint
2. Child's current social functioning, including at school academically, behaviourally, and in relationships with peers and staff
3. Personal and developmental history from pregnancy and delivery, including milestones, separations, physical illness, and temperamental style, e.g. emotionality, activity, sociability, and impulsivity
4. Family history
5. Information from observation of interviews with the family and child
6. Mental state
7. Physical examination
8. Investigations.

Children Act 1989

This emphasizes the 'supremacy of the interest of the child', i.e. that the child's safety is paramount. A Care or Supervision Order under this Act is taken out where a parent or parents cannot safely care for a child, i.e. on grounds of actual or serious risk of serious harm *and* this is attributable to the care. Objective current evidence carries more weight in court than predictions of experts.

☠ Safety issues

The Royal College of Psychiatrists[1] has issued important recommendations regarding safety issues when working with children and adolescents with mental disorders. In summary, these are:

• Children and young people with mental disorders can display significant violence and disinhibition, which could be directed towards the professionals who are trying to assess and provide treatment for them.
• Drugs and alcohol may be highly relevant aetiological factors in violent behaviour.
• Consider both the violence that the child may present and that presented by parents, who can become highly agitated, aggressive, and violent on behalf of their children, and whose violence can become exacerbated when there is parental disagreement, violence, separation, and major conflict.
• Family violence is an important backdrop to some violent behaviour by children and young people, and so one is often dealing with a broader context of significant intrafamilial violence.
• Similarly, mental disorder in children may be associated with significant parental mental disorder.
• Carrying weapons is on the increase among young people.

Reference

1 Royal College of Psychiatrists (2006). *Safety for Psychiatrists*. Council Report CR134. Royal College of Psychiatrists: London.

☠ Self-harm

Factors most likely to be associated with a higher risk of later suicide among adolescents who engage in self-harm behaviours include[1]

- Male gender
- Older age
- High suicidal intent
- Psychosis
- Depression
- Hopelessness
- Having an unclear reason for the act of deliberate self-harm.

The Royal College of Psychiatrists[1] recommends that:

- A consultant paediatrician and a consultant child and adolescent psychiatrist should be nominated as the joint service leaders for a service which looks after young people who deliberately harm themselves
- Admissions should generally be to a paediatric ward unless, for 14-to 16-year-olds, there exists a more suitable designated ward
- Agreement should be sought for the psychiatry assessment from the parent(s) or other adult(s) with parental responsibility
- In general, young people should remain in the overall care of a paediatrician
- The staff looking after the patient should have had training specifically orientated to work with young people and their families after deliberate self-harm, be skilled in risk assessment, and have consultation and supervision available to them.

Reference

1 Royal College of Psychiatrists (1998). *Managing Deliberate Self-harm in Young People*. Council Report CR64. Royal College of Psychiatrists: London.

☠ Child abuse

During the medical and psychological assessment of children and adolescents suspected of being victims of sexual or physical abuse/neglect, it is important to minimize physical and psychological trauma[1]. Types of child abuse include[2]:

- Physical abuse (non-accidental injury) such as bruises, fractures, wounds, and burns
- Sexual abuse
- Poisoning
- Suffocation
- Emotional neglect
- Munchausen's syndrome by proxy.

Wyatt and colleagues[2] have also summarized features of the medical history which should raise suspicion:

- Injuries inconsistent with the history given
- Injuries inappropriate for the developmental age
- Changing history of injury
- Vague history, lacking vivid details
- Delay in seeking medical attention
- Abnormal parental attitudes towards the child (e.g. apparent lack of concern)
- Frequent accident and emergency attendance.

The American Professional Society on the Abuse of Children[3] has issued practice guidelines for investigative interviewing in cases of alleged child abuse, which provide a useful framework:

- The child interview should take place as close to the time of the event as possible.
- An assessment of the child should determine if he or she is physically or mentally able to be interviewed at the time of presentation.
- Careful attention to safety concerns and the impact of delay of the interview process must be considered.
- The interview should take place in a neutral place…if possible. This will often be dictated by the acuteness of the presentation, e.g. a child who has been assaulted within the past 72 h should be seen in the emergency department. The setting should provide a safe place for the child to disclose this information.
- For some children, it is possible to obtain a comprehensive disclosure in one interview. In any case, it is necessary to conduct enough interviews (and only enough) to obtain a complete and accurate story. Repeated interviews of the child by different interviewers are discouraged and may compromise the integrity of the findings.
- Accurate documentation of the investigative interview must be maintained.
- To maintain consistency of the format and record of the interview, it is generally preferable to have one interviewer.
- The interview itself consists of introductions, rapport building, developmental screening, and competency check. In the latter, some states require that the interviewer establish if the child understands or can demonstrate the difference between the truth and a lie.

If there is any suspicion of child abuse, the case should be referred to a senior expert, such as a consultant paediatrician, a consultant in child and adolescent psychiatry or an accident and emergency consultant, who can arrange for the correct procedures, including an appropriate examination, to be carried out according to the local guidelines.

All mental health trusts in England and Wales now have child protection policies and a nominated consultant and/or senior nurse who should be informed of local issues.

Practical considerations when interviewing a case of suspected child abuse include:

- Avoid contamination of information
- Contact nominated child protection authorities for the area
- Facilitate safe and appropriate assessment, i.e. this may involve referral to appropriate authorities
- Consider informing social services
- Consider other practical issues such as risk of the child returning to the abusive situation.

References

1 Laraque D, DeMattia A, Low C (2006). Forensic child abuse evaluation: a review. *Mount Sinai Journal of Medicine* **73**: 1138–47.
2 Wyatt JP, Illingworth RN, Graham CA, Clancy MJ, Robertson CE (2006). *Oxford Handbook of Emergency Medicine,* 3rd edn. Oxford University Press: Oxford
3 American Professional Society on the Abuse of Children (2002). *Investigative interviewing in cases of alleged child abuse: practice guidelines.* American Professional Society on the Abuse of Children: Chicago, pp. 1–16.

Other psychiatric emergencies

Medical risks/complications in patients with eating disorders

With the dieting and progressive weight loss that occur in anorexia nervosa (owing to a morbid fear of fatness), various physical changes occur (Fig. 15.1) and result in a significantly increased mortality rate. This is six times greater than normal, with two-thirds being the result of starvation, and one-third due to suicide.

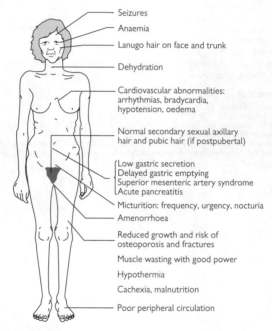

Seizures

Anaemia

Lanugo hair on face and trunk

Dehydration

Cardiovascular abnormalities: arrhythmias, bradycardia, hypotension, oedema

Normal secondary sexual axillary hair and pubic hair (if postpubertal)

Low gastric secretion
Delayed gastric emptying
Superior mesenteric artery syndrome
Acute pancreatitis

Micturition: frequency, urgency, nocturia

Amenorrhoea

Reduced growth and risk of osteoporosis and fractures

Muscle wasting with good power

Hypothermia

Cachexia, malnutrition

Poor peripheral circulation

Fig. 15.1 Physical features associated with anorexia nervosa. Reproduced from Puri BK, Laking PJ, Treasaden IH (2002). *Textbook of Psychiatry*, 2nd edn. Churchill Livingstone: Edinburgh.

In bulimia nervosa, in spite of a normal weight, extra medical complications occur in relation to self-induced vomiting, purging and/or diuretic abuse to counter the bingeing of food (Fig. 15.2).

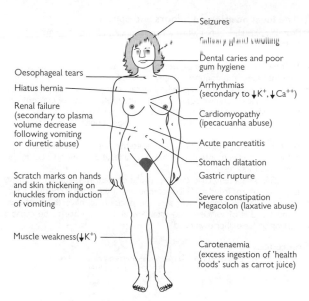

Fig. 15.2 Complications of vomiting, purging, and diuretic abuse. Reproduced from Puri BK, Laking PJ, Treasaden IH (2002). *Textbook of Psychiatry*, 2nd edn. Churchill Livingstone: Edinburgh.

① Psychotropic medication-related complications

Antidepressants should be started at low doses with close monitoring, although adult doses may be required. Methylphenidate for attention deficit hyperactivity disorder can cause depression and insomnia as well as growth retardation.

☼ Drug-induced states

① Risks involved in transition from child and adolescent services to adult services

Problems arise owing to a lack of integration between, and different values of, these services. Adult mental health services, largely geared to psychosis such as schizophrenia, may be unsuitable for adolescents and young adults, e.g. with conduct disorder, attention deficit hyperactivity disorder, or pervasive developmental disorders.

In addition, young people may be reluctant to take up help voluntarily from adult mental health services when not coerced to do so by parents, schools or professionals, e.g. social services.

① The legal position on minors and consent

- Professionals should not allow a person under 18 years to come to serious harm on the grounds that the minor and/or parents refuse consent to necessary and urgent treatment.
- 16- to 17-year-olds are presumed by statute to have capacity to give consent unless the contrary is demonstrated.
- A child under 16 years of age who has capacity (Gillick[1] competent—Common Law) can give consent, but, if they refuse, lack of consent can be over-ridden by those with parental responsibility or by a Court.
- It is unlikely that the Court will consider those under 13 years to have capacity.
- For children who are not Gillick-competent, those with parental responsibility give consent, but they have a legal obligation to act in the child's best interests.

A 'Gillick-competent' child can give a valid consent to medical treatment. A child may be regarded as 'Gillick-competent' if the doctor concludes that he or she has the capacity to make the decision to have the proposed treatment and is of sufficient understanding and intelligence to be capable of making up his or her own mind[2].

References

1 *Gillick v. West Norfolk and Wisbech Area Health Authority* [1986]. AC112.
2 Department of Health and Welsh office (1999). Mental Health Act 1983: Code of practice. The Stationery Office: London.

Psychiatric emergencies in people with learning disabilities

Presentation 260
Common medical problems 260
Other potential problems 260
Management 261

:⚙: Presentation

People with learning disabilities are increasingly in contact with healthcare professionals in accident and emergency units[1]. Their presentations may differ from those of non-learning disabled people owing to difficulties in communication, such as the following[2]:

- Aggression because of physical pain
- Self-injury as part of a mood disorder
- Epileptic seizures—more common in this group
- Head injury
- Deliberate self-harm
- Alcohol misuse.

References

1 Sowney M, Barr OG (2006). Caring for adults with intellectual disabilities: perceived challenges for nurses in accident and emergency units. *Journal of Advanced Nursing* **55**: 36–45.
2 Royal College of Psychiatrists (2004). *Psychiatric Services to Accident and Emergency Departments.* Council Report CR118. Royal College of Psychiatrists: London.

① Common medical problems

The following medical problems are particularly common in patients with learning disabilities (partly after Sowney and Barr, 2006[1]):

- Respiratory disease
- Gastrointestinal reflux disease
- *Helicobacter pylori* infection
- Dental disease
- Thyroid/other hormonal dysfunction
- Early dementia
- Increased risk of trauma, falls, accidents, and death as a result of:
  - Sensory impairment
  - Epilepsy
  - Osteoporosis
  - Polypharmacy.

Reference

1 Sowney M, Barr OG (2006). Caring for adults with intellectual disabilities: perceived challenges for nurses in accident and emergency units. *Journal of Advanced Nursing* **55**: 36–45.

:☠: Other potential problems

- Abuse
- Neglect
- Sexually inappropriate behaviour.

① Management

Guidelines to management include:
- Gather information from all relevant informants
- Consider recent life events and the patient's current situation
- Assess the patient from a developmental perspective
- In the differential diagnosis consider whether the behaviour is normative
- Reassure the patient by involving people with whom they are familiar
- Avoid high doses of medication
- If medications are appropriate, consider doses carefully. A lower dose of medication may be safer, in view of increased risks of side-effects.
- Use the least restrictive intervention methods possible.

The Royal College of Psychiatrists[1] have issued the following guidance on looking after people with learning disability who present in an accident and emergency department:
- Always believe what the person tells you in the absence of contrary evidence.
- Offer appropriate treatment for the presenting problem as required.
- Consider the issue of consent to treatment and facilitate the person in providing valid consent. Use simple language, pictures and diagrams, such as that used in the Books Beyond Words series[2].
- With the person's consent, involve the social network, e.g. family member or the carer from the community home.

The recommendations of the Royal College of Psychiatrists[1] include:
- Assess for physical illness. Treat on clinical need without discrimination. Consult and involve the person in the care you intend to provide.
- Use simple language when taking a history, and when explaining investigations and treatment. Seek the person's consent for investigations.
- Consider the role of carers/supporters in assisting the person to give a history. Carers can facilitate understanding of your care plan.
- Avoid medication to control aggressive behaviour. Make use of a low-stimulation environment.
- Where concern for the person's mental health is present, liaise with the local community mental health team for people with learning disability.
- If abuse or exploitation of the person is suspected, refer to the local social services department and their policy on vulnerable adults.
- Ensure follow-up through liaison with the general practitioner.

References

1 Royal College of Psychiatrists (2004). *Psychiatric Services to Accident and Emergency Departments*. Council Report CR118. Royal College of Psychiatrists: London.
2 Hollins S, Bernal J, Gregory M, Redmond D (1998). *Books Beyond Words*. St George's Hospital Medical School and Gaskell Press: London.

Emergencies in old-age psychiatry

Presentation of psychiatric disorders 264
Accident and emergency departments 266
Medication 268
Discharge from accident and emergency departments 271
General management issues in old-age psychiatry 272
Driving 272

The nature of emergencies in old-age psychiatry will vary with the source of referral. In those over 65 years of age in the community, the most common psychiatric disorders are neuroses and personality disorder, followed by depression and dementia. Of those referred to old-age psychiatric services, the most common psychiatric disorders are dementia, acute confusional state, and depression. In general medical wards the most common emergencies are acute confusional states, which may be superimposed on dementia.

① Presentation of psychiatric disorders

Psychiatric disorders presenting as an emergency in old-age psychiatry include primary psychiatric disorders and psychiatric problems secondary to underlying medical illnesses.

The presentation of psychiatric disorders in the elderly may differ from that in younger adults. Importantly, atypical ways in which depression may present in the elderly include[1]:

• Agitated depression—in contrast to the retardation more commonly seen in younger patients
• Symptoms masked by concurrent physical illness
• A minimization or denial of low mood and/or suicidal ideation
• Hypochondriasis
• Complaints of loneliness
• Physical complaints disproportionate to organic pathology
• Pain of unknown origin
• Onset of neurotic symptoms
• Depressive pseudodementia
• Substance misuse, especially alcohol
• Accidents.

Psychiatric problems can result from, or impact on, underlying medical illnesses. For example, dementia can lead to an increased risk of hypothermia, and medical illnesses can lead to an acute confusional state.

It can be difficult to differentiate between delirium and dementia, and indeed the two may be comorbid (see below).

Delusional disorders (paraphrenia) may occur in elderly patients, particularly those who[1]:

• Live alone
• Suffer from sensory deprivation, for example resulting from
    • Poor eyesight
    • Hearing difficulties.

Reference

1 Puri BK, Laking PJ, Treasaden IH (2002). *Textbook of Psychiatry*, 2nd edn. Churchill Livingstone: Edinburgh.

:O: Accident and emergency departments

The Royal College of Psychiatrists[1] makes the points shown in Table 17.1 regarding the assessment and management of elderly patients with psychiatric problems who present in accident and emergency departments.

Table 17.1 Assessment and management of the elderly with mental health problems in accident and emergency departments. Reproduced with kind permission of Royal College of Psychiatrists[1]

- Mental health problems may present differently in older people. For example, depression may present with pronounced physical symptoms such as pain

- Difficulties in obtaining high-quality information in the presence of cognitive impairment due to delirium or dementia, both commonly encountered in accident and emergency departments

- Differentiation between delirium, dementia, and comorbid delirium and dementia. These two syndromes have different aetiologies and management strategies, with the presence of delirium pointing towards an underlying physical cause

- The high levels of cognitive impairment, with associated behaviour such as wandering, may be problematic in a busy accident and emergency department

- The greater impact of a changing environment on those with cognitive impairment or sensory impairment

- The frequent presence of comorbid physical and psychiatric illness. It may be difficult to distinguish the relative importance of symptoms, such as weight loss or apathy, when two or more processes may be occurring simultaneously and presentations can represent a wide variety of different types of pathology. Older people who present with memory problems, lack of concentration, anxiety, and apparent disorientation could have had a recent myocardial infraction, a urinary tract infection or a severe depressive illness.

- The frequent presence of multiple physical illnesss, which may limit treatment options because of drug intereactions or contraindictions

- Communication problems when an individual has sensory impairment

- The effects of prescribed and over-the-counter medications, particularly with polypharmacy

- The different social supports and social networks that older people have

- The different psychiatric services provided for working age adult and older people

If an elderly patient appears to have a communication problem, then its nature should be assessed[1] (Table 17.2).

Table 17.2 Communication problems in the elderly. Reproduced with kind permission of Royal College of Psychiatrists[1]

- Is there a hearing problem?
- Is there a language difficulty?
- Is it the clinician that does not understand the patient and is therefore making assumptions about their cognitive state?
- Does the patient understand the clinician' questions?
- If so, what type of questions is understood, and what type is not understood?
- Is there a problem in concentration?
- Is there a problem with registration?
- Is there a problem with memory?
- Is the patient orientated?
- Is there a dyspraxia?
- Are there any problems with speech, and if so, of what type?
- Is there any perseveration?

Reference

1 Royal College of Psychiatrists (2004). *Psychiatric Services to Accident and Emergency Departments.* Council Report CR118. Royal College of Psychiatrists: London.

ⓘ Medication

The pharmacokinetics of many drugs differ in the elderly compared with younger adults. Compared with the latter, in general the elderly have[1]:

- A reduced total body mass
- A reduced proportion of total body water
- A reduced proportion of muscle tissue
- An increased proportion of adipose tissue
- Different plasma concentrations of proteins—often a reduced level of plasma albumin and an increased level of plasma gamma globulin, for example
- Reduced hepatic metabolism
- Reduced glomerular filtration rate
- Reduced renal clearance.

Therefore, the side-effects of medication taken by elderly patients need to be carefully considered before prescription; for example, those that cause postural hypotension (such as antipsychotics and tricyclic antidepressants) may cause an elderly patient to fall and suffer a fracture[2]. Polypharmacy is more common in the elderly, and can increase the risk of side-effects. The elderly are also more sensitive to sedatives and anxiolytics, with an increased risk of postural instability, hangover sedation, and impaired cognitive and psychomotor performance.

There are risks associated with over-or under-medication in treating agitation. The physical condition, including liver, kidney, and heart functioning, needs to be assessed and current medications borne in mind because of the risk of adverse interactions. Treatment should be with the lowest effective doses. Medication should be introduced slowly and carefully to avoid side-effects and increase compliance. Small quantities of medication should be prescribed at a time. Carers and relatives should be advised and encouraged to be involved in monitoring medication compliance.

Atypical antipsychotics should be used with caution in the elderly, in addition to their recognized relative contraindications in those with a history of cardiovascular disease or epilepsy. Olanzapine and risperidone have been associated with an increased risk of stroke in elderly patients with dementia. The UK *Committee on Safety of Medicines* have issued the following advice:

- Olanzapine should not be used for treating behavioural symptoms of dementia
- Olanzapine is not licensed for acute psychoses in the elderly
- The possibility of cerebrovascular events should be considered carefully before treating any patient with a history of stroke or transient ischaemic attack; risk factors for cerebrovascular disease (e.g. hypertension, diabetes, smoking, and atrial fibrillation) should also be considered.

Lewy body dementia (seen in Parkinson's disease) may have pre-existing mild extrapyramidal features. Such individuals may have extreme sensitivity to the extrapyramidal side-effects of antipsychotic medication.

An algorithm from the Royal College of Psychiatrists[3] for the sedation of elderly patients is shown Fig. 17.1.

Older adults

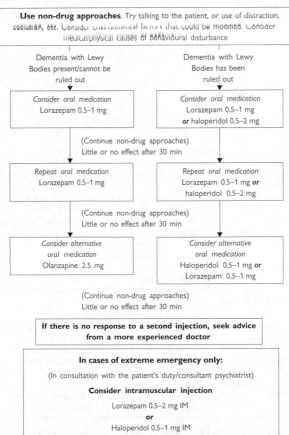

Use non-drug approaches. Try talking to the patient, or use of distraction, seclusion, etc. Consider environmental factors that could be modified. Consider medical/physical causes of behavioural disturbance

Dementia with Lewy
Bodies present/cannot be
ruled out

Dementia with Lewy
Bodies has been
ruled out

Consider oral medication
Lorazepam 0.5–1 mg

Consider oral medication
Lorazepam 0.5–1 mg
or haloperidol 0.5–2 mg

(Continue non-drug approaches)
Little or no effect after 30 min

Repeat oral medication
Lorazepam 0.5–1 mg

Repeat oral medication
Lorazepam 0.5–1 mg *or*
haloperidol 0.5–2 mg

(Continue non-drug approaches)
Little or no effect after 30 min

*Consider alternative
oral medication*
Olanzapine 2.5 mg

*Consider alternative
oral medication*
Haloperidol 0.5–1 mg *or*
Lorazepam 0.5–1 mg

(Continue non-drug approaches)
Little or no effect after 30 min

**If there is no response to a second injection, seek advice
from a more experienced doctor**

In cases of extreme emergency only:

(In consultation with the patient's duty/consultant psychiatrist)

Consider intramuscular injection

Lorazepam 0.5–2 mg IM

or

Haloperidol 0.5–1 mg IM

(only use haloperidol if dementia with Lewy Bodies has been ruled out)

Fig. 17.1 Sedation guidelines for accident and emergency departments for elderly patients. Reproduced with kind permission of the Royal College of Psychiatrists[3].

These guidelines apply where a frail patient over 65 years of age is behaving in a disturbed or violent manner that is unusual for him/her and that cannot be modified by interventions already in their care-plan. For physically fit patients and those currently/previously treated with higher doses of antipsychotics, the protocol for younger adults may be more appropriate. Details of the clinical situation and all interventions must be recorded in the patient's medical notes.

Emergency resuscitation equipment, procyclidine injection and flumazenil injection must be available before treatment
Medication should be the last resort in older people. If required, medication must be used cautiously and only by the oral route (except in very extreme emergencies—see lower panel**). (Note the Mental Health Act 1983 status of the patient.)

Monitoring of the patient must be performed and recorded according to the guidelines below after any injection is given.

Procyclidine injection 5–10 mg can be given iv or im for acute dystonic or parkinsonian reactions.

Flumazenil (a benzodiazepine antagonist) must be given if the respiration rate falls to <10 breaths/min after lorazepam has been used (see panel below).

Give flumazenil 200 mcg IV over 15 s. If the desired level of consciousness is not obtained within 60 s, a further 100 mcg can be injected and repeated at 60 s intervals to a maximum total dose of 1 mg (1000 mcg) in 24 h (initial + eight additional doses). Monitor respiration rate continuosly until it returns to baseline level.

NB. The effect of flumazenil may wear off and respiratory depression can return—monitoring must therefore continue beyond initial recovery of respiratiory function.

Example of a monitoring schedule
After injections, this monitoring schedule must be followed, unless there are compelling reasons for doing otherwise, and must be recorded in all cases:
• Pulse and respiration as soon as possible after injection, then every 5 min for 1 h
• Temperature (using Tempadots) as soon as possilble after injection as a baseline, then at 5, 10, 15, and 60 min
• Blood pressure at 30 and 60 min after injection
• Monitor for signs of neurological reactions (e.g. acute dystonia, acute parkinsonism).
If not followed, the 'responsible nurse' must document the reasons why.

Fig. 17.1 (*Contd.*) Sedation guidelines for accident and emergency departments for elderly patients. Reproduced with kind permission from the Royal College of Psychiatrists[3].

References

1 Puri BK (2006a). *Drugs in Psychiatry*. Oxford University Press: Oxford.
2 Puri BK, Laking PJ, Treasaden IH (2002). *Textbook of Psychiatry*, 2nd edn. Churchill Livingstone: Edinburgh.
3 Royal College of Psychiatrists (2004). *Psychiatric Services to Accident and Emergency Departments*. Council Report CR118. Royal College of Psychiatrists: London.

① Discharge from accident and emergency departments

Elderly patients are more vulnerable following discharge from emergency departments because of their multiple pathologies and atypical symptoms. Risk indicators include:

- Previous medical history
- Pre-admission status, e.g. dementia
- Unsuitable or changed social circumstances
- Living alone
- Lack of family or social support
- Recent bereavement
- Difficulty with mobility
- Unsuitable home circumstances, e.g. stairs
- Financial management difficulties, e.g. for food, heating
- Evidence of inability to cope at home
- Poor personal hygiene, cleanliness, unsuitable clothing
- Weight loss
- Shortness of breath
- Impaired mobility
- History of repeated falls: are these caused by
  - External factors that could be corrected, e.g. loose carpets, poor lighting, unsuitable footwear?
  - Internal factors such as cerebrovascular disease, arthritis, side-effects of medication or need for walking frame?

If uncertainty remains in spite of an elderly person saying they can cope alone at home, consult relatives, the community services, and general practitioner.

Consider occupational therapy and/or physiotherapy assessments, if appropriate, at the patient's home. This may result in recommendations for equipment and adaptations.

Mobilize community services, e.g. district nurse, health visitor, home help, social worker.

Safe discharge home remains the goal, as hospitalization can lead to confusion, disorientation, and fear in the elderly.

General management issues in old-age psychiatry

- Early comprehensive assessment of medical, psychiatric, and social aspects
- Assess at home, and interview relatives and carers
- Keep patient at home as long as possible. This reduces confusion
- There is a need to consider the carer, who may be elderly and ill as well
- Consideration of settings for management, e.g. warden-controlled flats, residential or nursing homes, psychiatric hospital
- Involvement of other services, e.g. community psychiatric nurse, social worker. Practical help, e.g. home help.
- However, families remain the most important source of support and need support themselves, including to counter their established high rates of physical and psychiatric illness
- Carer-related issues are often an important focus of management in old-age psychiatry, especially when there are doubts as to the physical/mental health of the primary carer. This may need to be adequately addressed by assessment and referral within a community team
- Consider safety issues, such as mobility, use of fire and gas, domestic appliances.

⊕ Driving

- Many people with early dementia are capable of driving. The risk of crashes is low for the first 3 years after onset of dementia. In the UK, the Driving and Vehicle Licensing Authority (DVLA) must be notified of all new cases diagnosed with Alzheimer's disease or other dementias
- Doctors must make, on interviewing the patient, an immediate assessment of safety to drive and notify the DVLA, if necessary without the patient's consent, if the patient is assessed as unsafe to drive
- Cognitive testing is a poor predictor of driving ability.

Emergencies in psychiatry in primary care

Epidemiology 274
Range of cases seen in primary care compared to
     psychiatric practice 275
Neurotic and stress-related disorders 276
Safety considerations 282

Epidemiology

- The majority of psychiatric patients are dealt with by their GPs and not by psychiatrists. Epidemiological studies in the community have indicated that for about every 1 000 of the population:
  - One-quarter, 250, have psychiatric morbidity
  - Of these, about 230 (90%) consult their general practitioner.
- The GP identifies psychiatric morbidity in only about two-thirds of such cases.
- Of those the GP identifies, he will treat most himself.
- Less than one-tenth of cases identified by a GP will be referred to specialist psychiatric services.
- Less than a third of these will receive inpatient psychiatric care, i.e. less than 1% of the total population, and only 2.5% of those with psychiatric morbidity in the community.
- It has been estimated that in an average general practice population of 2500:
  - Three hundred will have neurotic and stress-related disorders.
  - About 55 will be chronically mentally ill.
  - Thirty will have chronic alcoholism, of which the GP is aware of only five.
  - Twelve will have severe depressive disorder.
  - Ten individuals will have learning disability.
  - There will be one parasuicide act a year.
  - There will be one suicide every 3 years.

⊙ Range of cases seen in primary care compared to psychiatric practice

- A common difference between psychiatric emergencies presenting to the GP as opposed to those seen by a psychiatrist is the presence in the cases of GPs of physical symptoms, physical illness, and/or fear of physical illness complicating the psychiatric presentation.
- Where physical and psychiatric disorders coexist, the risk is that GPs may focus on the management of the overt physical disorder alone.
- Up to one in four new consultations to GPs present with physical problems for which no physical cause is found. (This is in fact lower than for general medical new outpatient consultations, especially for cardiology, gastroenterology, and neurology clinics, where rates may reach 30–50%.)
- The hidden psychiatric morbidity, i.e. those with psychiatric symptoms not identified by a GP, is frequently diagnosed as suffering from minor physical conditions.
- The whole range of psychiatric emergencies may be seen by a GP. Particularly common are:
  - Depression, often reactive to current stressors, albeit in a vulnerable personality
  - Panic attacks
  - Suicidal behaviour
  - Stupor
  - Acute stress (situational) reaction
  - Bereavement reactions
  - Confusion in the elderly
  - Bizarre behaviour
  - Histrionic behaviour (over-emotional, over-dramatic, etc.), often caused by personality disorder
  - Alcohol-related problems
  - Violence
  - Emergencies arising from domestic crises, including domestic violence and in 'problem families'.
- It is important to exclude non-psychiatric causes of emergency presentations, e.g. physical illness without cerebral involvement, law involvement, problems in others, e.g. family, carers, friends, over-anxiety in others, including professionals.
- Compared to cases referred to psychiatrists, severe psychotic mental illness such as schizophrenia, self-harm, and drug abuse are less common.
- GPs' knowledge of their patients can lead to their picking up early prodromal changes associated with the onset of psychoses such as schizophrenia. For example, there may be subtle changes in the way in which the patient interacts with their GP.
- Alcohol abuse will often compound psychiatric presentations to GPs.
- Patients may also frequently demand immediate relief of symptoms, in particular by medication.

⊙ Neurotic and stress-related disorders

Concept of neurosis

- Neurosis is a general term for a group of mental illnesses in which anxiety, phobic, obsessional, and hypochondriacal symptoms predominate. The dominant symptom determines the formal diagnosis, but several commonly coexist.
- Neurotic symptoms differ from normal symptoms such as anxiety only by their intensity, not qualitatively.
- Neuroses are abnormal psychogenic (psychologically-caused) reactions.
- Most neuroses are precipitated by normal life stressors and are often associated with a vulnerable personality disorder, especially dependent and anankastic (obsessional) personality disorders.
- Neurosis is twice as common in women as in men.

Factors associated with development of neurotic and stress-related disorders

- Lower social class
- Unemployment
- Divorced, separated or widowed
- Renting rather than owning own home
- No educational qualifications
- Urban rather than rural.
  (NB. The homeless and prisoners have twice the risk of the general population.)

Anxiety disorders

- Anxiety is a normal mood and, like pain, a warning sign
- Anxiety is accompanied by bodily (somatic) symptoms due to Cannon's (adrenergic) fight or flight reaction
- Primary generalized anxiety disorder is rare compared to mixed anxiety and depressive disorder
- Anxiety is more often associated with other psychiatric disorders, such as depression, than generalized anxiety disorder, especially when the onset is after the age of 35 years
- Cognitive therapy and anxiety management techniques are effective treatments for generalized anxiety disorder

Benzodiazepines should not be prescribed as hypnotics for more than 10 nights, or as anxiolytics for more than 4 weeks, owing to the risk of dependency.

Table 18.1 Frequency of neurotic conditions

Condition	Frequency (%)
Mixed anxiety and depression	48
Generalized anxiety disorder	28
Depression	14
Phobia	12
Obsessive-compulsive disorder	10
Panic disorder	6

Table 18.2 Psychological features of generalized anxiety disorder

Symptoms	Characteristics
Psychic	• Feelings of threat and foreboding • Difficulty in concentrating or 'mind going blank' • Distractible • Feeling keyed up, on edge, tense or unable to relax • Early insomnia and nightmares • Irritability • Noise intolerance (e.g. of children or music)
Panic attacks	• Unexpected severe acute exacerbations of psychic and somatic anxiety symptoms with intense fear or discomfort • Not triggered by situations • Individuals cannot 'sit out' the attack
Other features	• Lability of mood • Depersonalization (dreamlike sensation of unreality of self or part of self) • Hypnagogic and hypnopompic hallucinations (when, respectively, going off to or waking from sleep) • Perceptual distortion (e.g. distortion of walls or the sound of other people talking)

Table 18.3 Differential diagnosis between generalized anxiety and depressive disorders

Generalized anxiety disorder	Depressive disorder
• Common in early adult life	• Commoner in later adult life
• Onset age 20–40 years	• Onset age 20–60+ years
• More frequent in those of premorbid anxious personality	• More frequent in those of previous stable personality
• Previous episodes of anxiety	• Previous episodes of depression or even mania
• Panic attacks frequent	• Panic attacks rare
• Lack of concentration	• Loss of interest (anhedonia)
• Minor loss of appetite	• Major loss of appetite or increased appetite
• Sexual performance reduced	• Reduced libido
• No diurnal variation of mood	• Marked diurnal variation of mood
• Initial insomnia	• Early morning wakening
• Somatic symptoms common	• Ideas of reference, guilt, and hopelessness common
• More related to external precipitants	• Less frequently related to external precipitants
• Chronic course	• Episodic course

NB. Diagnostic category of neurosis often changes over time and in medical record; 90% of individuals with neurosis are labelled neurotic depression.

Disorders which can present primarily with symptoms of anxiety

- Generalized anxiety disorder
- Panic disorder
- Phobic disorders
- Obsessive-compulsive disorder
- Depressive disorder
- Schizophrenia and other paranoid psychosis
- Early dementia (e.g. catastrophic reactions upon psychometric testing)
- Ictal anxiety due to epilepsy, especially temporal lobe epilepsy
- Thyrotoxicosis
- Phaeochromocytoma
- Unexpressed complaints of physical illness (e.g. lump in breast)
- Drug and alcohol abuse, dependency, and withdrawal symptoms (e.g. delirium tremens, caffeinism).

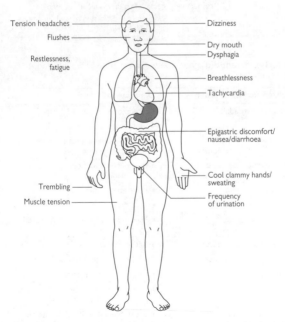

Fig. 18.1 Somatic Clinical features of generalized anxiety disorder. Reproduced from Puri BK, Laking PJ, Treasaden IH (2002). *Textbook of Psychiatry*, 2nd edn. Churchill Livingstone: Edinburgh.

Panic disorder

- Panic attacks are discrete periods of intense fear or discomfort caused by acute psychic and somatic anxiety symptoms, which are unexpected and not triggered by situations.
- Panic disorder is effectively treated by cognitive behavioural approaches.
- Antidepressants, especially the SSRIs and clomipramine, are also beneficial in panic disorder.

Mixed anxiety and depressive disorder

- A diagnosis of mixed anxiety and depressive disorder is made when symptoms of both anxiety and depression are present, but neither condition is severe enough to justify a separate diagnosis.
- The term neurosis does not now include depression if this is the predominant symptom. It is instead classified under mood (affective) disorders as a depressive episode.

Phobic disorders

- Fear is a normal prudent situational anxiety.
- A phobia is an inappropriate situational anxiety with avoidance.
- Specific (isolated) phobia, such as of animals, is the most common, but agoraphobia, a fear not only of open spaces but of crowds and difficulty in making an easy escape, is most seen by psychiatrists.
- Exposure techniques are the psychological treatment of choice and may involve homework assignments.
- MAOI antidepressants such as phenelzine specifically relieve symptoms of agoraphobia and social phobia.

Table 18.4 Age of onset, sex, ratio, characteristics, and treatment response of phobias

	Specific phobias	Agoraphobia	Social phobia
Age of onset	In childhood 3–8 years M = F	15–30 years F 2.5 : 1 M	In children under 5 years, and puberty to 35 years F 2.5 : 1 M
Feared objects	Animals (zoophobia) Thunder (tonitophobia) Heights (acrophobia) Spiders (arachnophobia) Bees (apiphobia) Birds (orniphobia)	*Classic symptoms* Open spaces Crowded places Main roads Public transport Housebound syndrome *Also,* situations from which escape is difficult, e.g. a bus between stops, the middle seats in a row at the cinema, a supermarket queue	Formal social occasions Eating in public Talking socially Situations in which one feels under social scrutiny, e.g. talking in small groups, eating in front of others
Behaviour therapy	+++	+	++
SSRI and MAOI anti-depressants	—	+	+

Table 18.5 Differential diagnosis of social phobia and depression

	Social phobia	Depression
Loss of interest (anhedonia)	—	+
Energy	Normal	Reduced

Table 18.6 Differential diagnosis of general social phobia and panic disorder

	General social phobia	**Panic disorder**
Panic attacks	In feared social situation	Unpredictable
Fear	Appearing foolish or awkward	Losing control or death
Social encounter if with friends	Little difference	Can enjoy

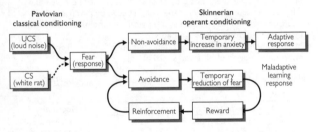

Fig. 18.2 Behavioural learning theory and the development of Phobias. Reproduced from Puri BK, Laking PJ, Treasaden IH (2002). *Textbook of Psychiatry*, 2nd edn. Churchill Livingstone: Edinburgh.

Obsessive-compulsive disorder

- Non-situational preoccupation with subjective compulsion despite conscious resistance.
- Can be thoughts (ruminations/obsessions), although ruminations alone may be insufficient for the diagnosis, or acts (rituals/compulsions).
- Insight is maintained: 'It's silly but I can't stop it', or at least individuals recognize that the thought or image is their own and they have generated it.
- Obsessional symptoms are common in depressive disorder, and any depressive component should always be adequately treated.
- Behaviour therapy treatments include thought stopping for ruminations and response prevention for rituals.
- SSRIs and clomipramine specifically treat obsessional symptoms.

Post-traumatic stress disorder

- A reaction of normal individuals to a major trauma.
- Intrusive recollections, emotional numbing, increased autonomic arousal, and hypervigilance occur. Diagnostic criteria are given in Chapter 5.
- Meetings of groups of survivors and critical incident debriefing within 1–2 days may be preventative.
- Self-help and mutual support groups are helpful.
- Psychological treatments include rehearsal of the 'trauma story', such as 'testimony'.
- Antidepressant drugs are effective, although their main effect may be on the associated depressed mood.

ⓘ Safety considerations

- GPs see psychiatric emergencies not only in the surgery but in the patient's home.
- The presence of a relative or friend may assist in providing independent information and corroboration of the patient's condition. Patients may, however, wish to be seen alone and may fear the GP may be biased by the presence and opinions of others present.
- Clearly, the GP needs to be aware of the risks of undertaking home visits alone, particularly to known uncooperative and potentially aggressive patients, but also to all new or relatively unknown patients. It is important to consider the risks before undertaking such a visit and, if in doubt, such a visit should be conducted with a colleague. An added safety measure before undertaking domiciliary visits is to let colleagues know of your movements and who and where you are seeing individual patients to enable them to alert others to assist if you fail to make contact within a reasonable time.
- Patients may be hostile and refuse to open the door to domiciliary visits, particularly when paranoid. Persistence by the GP may be required, including via discussions through the letterbox. If admission to the home is refused or no answer is obtained, consideration may need to be given to undertaking a formal Mental Health Act assessment regarding the individual's detainability in conjunction with an Approved Social Worker, and, if considered prudent, police back-up.
- Power of entry to a home and removal of the patient to a place of safety can be authorized under section 135 of the Mental Health Act 1983 on the grounds of mental disorder for the patient's health, safety or because of risk to others, by application to a magistrate. To enter a home without the owner's permission is otherwise trespass.
- GPs and others should resist the temptation to transport psychiatric patients to hospital in their own car because of the risks of the patient becoming agitated in the car or attempting to leave or, indeed, jumping from the car, which itself may be uninsured for such purposes.
- The decision as to whether a patient requires inpatient treatment may depend less on the severity of their psychiatric symptoms, e.g. auditory hallucinations, than on the support, including from family, available to that individual if he remains at home, i.e. family and/or social factors may be an important determining factor in admission.

Assertive outreach, crisis resolution and intensive home treatment teams, and early intervention services

Assertive outreach *285*
Crisis resolution and intensive home treatment teams *288*
Early intervention services *290*

- The specialist psychiatric services described in this chapter represent developments which, in the UK, have supplemented community mental health teams, which themselves followed the move to more community-based mental health services from the old asylums. They are sometimes referred to as Modernization Teams, as described in the UK Department of Health Mental Health Policy Implementation Guide of 2001. Although the new services are clearly defined in this document, there is much variation in terminology and practice.

- In the USA assertive outreach is referred to as assertive community treatment (ACT). Such services of high standard in the USA are sometimes referred to as Programme for ACT (PACT).

- In Europe services that followed this model but often lacked features of its structure, such as shared caseloads and extended hours, are referred to as Intensive Case Management Teams. In the USA, the work of The Department of Veterans' Affairs ACT teams are also called Intensive Psychiatric Community Care.

- ACT crossed the Atlantic to the UK following demonstrated effectiveness in early studies. The original model programme was a community follow-up service which attempted to sustain life outside hospital through skills training and was referred to as Training in Community Living. The effect of training, however, was demonstrated to wear off.

- A classic randomized control trial[1] showed that a community follow-up service reduced hospitalization, symptomatology, and improved social outcomes, including social stability and housing.

Reference

1 Stein LI, Test MA (1980). Alternative to mental hospital treatment, 1. Conceptual model, treatment progress and clinical evaluations. *Archives of General Psychiatry* **37**: 392–7.

① Assertive outreach

- Developed from the US ACT and the modernization team most widely implemented in the UK, Assertive Outreach services, are characterized by:
  - Small caseload size with a focus on severe mental illness alone.
  - A blurring of the traditional roles of mental health professionals.
  - Emphasis on sustained efforts to follow-up previously poorly compliant patients actively.
  - Low patient-to-staff ratios (10:1 up to 15:1).
  - Frequency of contact, which often takes place at the patient's home, is high, is adjusted to need, and ranges from daily to once a fortnight, but characteristically is about twice a week.
  - Intended to be easily accessible at times of crisis.
  - Not time-limited.
- Assertive outreach interventions concentrate on:
  - Developing long-term therapeutic relationships with previously hard-to-engage patients.
  - Intense monitoring of symptoms and subsequent rapid adjustment of treatments if required.
  - Medication may be administered by staff daily if needed.
- Non-medical interventions include:
  - Intensive emotional and/or practical support.
  - Specific psychological interventions, such as problem-solving or cognitive behavioural therapy.
  - Family work and support for carers.

The effectiveness of assertive outreach

- This has been much researched, although there have been differences in the interpretations of results. Much of the research was undertaken in the USA where community psychiatric services were relatively poorly developed compared to the UK, and thus perhaps excessively favoured assertive outreach services.
- A Cochrane database meta-analysis of the evidence base[1] demonstrated that assertive outreach resulted in:
  - Better engagement of patients than with routine care.
  - Reduced both the rate of admission to hospital and the total time in hospital.
  - Improved patient satisfaction and housing and employment stability.
- There was, however, no difference in symptoms detected on mental state examination or in measures of social functioning between those in receipt of assertive outreach and those in receipt of standard care.
- Further review of the evidence in 2001 by Bond and colleagues[2], in which the outcomes of 25 studies of ACT were reviewed, showed that assertive outreach did have:
  - A large impact in retaining individuals in treatment, reducing hospital use, and improving housing.
  - A moderate impact on symptoms and the quality of life.
  - A weak impact on social functioning, employment, substance misuse, offending, and imprisonment.

- Assertive outreach is a tertiary psychiatric service, accepting referrals from community mental health teams, and is a way of organizing mental health services and targeting a difficult-to-engage severely mentally ill population rather than a new treatment approach.
- Of studies of assertive outreach in the UK that have failed to demonstrate effectiveness over standard care, the PRISM study[3] compared intensive community care with standard care and found no significant differences in effectiveness. In fact, intensive care appeared to worsen the prognosis for those who were mild and moderately handicapped. In the UK700 studies, in which intensive case management with low caseloads was compared with standard care, significant benefits were demonstrated.
- While it has been argued that assertive outreach may not provide significant benefits to standard UK community mental health services owing to the latter's superiority over US community mental health services, criticisms of studies in the UK based on whether there was 'fidelity to the assertive outreach model' have questioned the findings of studies not demonstrating benefit. For instance, in the UK700 studies, a multidisciplinary team approach was not adopted.

References

1 Marshall M, Lockwood A (1998). Assertive community treatment for people with severe mental disorders. *Cochrane Library* **2**: 1–32.

2 Bond GR, Drake RE, Mueser KT, Latimer E (2001). Assertive community treatment for people with severe mental illness: critical ingredients and impact on patients. *Disease Management and Health Outcomes* **9**: 141–59.

3 Phelan M, Strathdee G, Thornicroft G (eds) (1995). *Emergency Mental Health Services in the Community.* Cambridge University Press: Cambridge.

⊙ Crisis resolution and intensive home treatment teams

- Within the UK the terms crisis resolution team, crisis assessment and treatment team, and intensive home treatment team are frequently used synonymously.
- The origins of such teams relate to a few assertive community treatment trials in the USA which had home treatment components and a classic study undertaken in Sydney, Australia, by Hoult and others[1], which reported in 1986 on the use of a crisis team for the mentally ill.
- An earlier term, crisis intervention team, however, related to the application of crisis intervention theory, not necessarily with the focus of preventing admission to psychiatric hospital.
- The focus for crisis resolution teams has been to reduce the need for acute psychiatric hospital admissions and occupancy of beds. To achieve this the teams characteristically assess all patients being considered for emergency admission and, if practically possible, avoid admission by initiating intensive home treatment until the crisis is resolved.
- Such teams have also been used to reduce the length of inpatient stay by facilitating early discharge with intensive home treatment and support.
- While assertive outreach teams provide long-term community care to a severely mentally ill group, crisis resolution teams intervene over a shorter period and with a much wider range of diagnoses.
- Crisis resolution teams, while separate from community mental health teams, are:
  - Multidisciplinary
  - Focused on those emergency situations where admission would otherwise be indicated
  - Like assertive outreach, crisis resolution teams have lower patient-to-staff ratios, with a capacity to visit even up to several times a day, with 24-h availability, and response within 1 h when possible. There may be direct administration of medication up to 4 times daily if required
  - Review patient's progress at least daily
  - Have a gate-keeping role, so that no individuals are admitted to an acute psychiatric inpatient unit without the crisis resolution team assessing the patient first and considering whether intensive home support and treatment would avoid hospital admission
  - Usually patients are only under the care of crisis resolution teams for less than 2 months.
- Interventions follow standard psychiatric practice with:
  - A comprehensive initial assessment followed by standard medication and psychosocial interventions
  - Emphasize treatment in the community as an alternative to that in hospital.

- Some such services have wider goals, including variations in emphasis on fundamental longer-term change and service user involvement.
- Service users usually welcome the use of crisis resolution teams.
- However, the evidence base is limited and sometimes contradictory, especially as to which patients are most successfully managed by such an approach.
- The advantage of separate crisis resolution teams is that staff are dedicated to the management of emergencies and not otherwise diverted by other priorities. They attract staff enthused by such an approach who then in turn gain extensive experience in such work. Such intensive work on a sustained basis can, however, be associated with staff burnout.
- An alternative approach is to integrate crisis resolution teams with community mental health teams. This has advantages in terms of continuity of care, i.e. the same staff will manage the patient in all settings, and the facilitation of care planning.
- Good psychiatric practice should emphasize early detection of onset of deterioration in mental state and intervention appropriately at that stage. In contrast, it is of note that crisis resolution teams only become involved when deterioration has taken place and is severe.
- There is little evidence for the benefits of intensive home treatment teams after about 6 months.

Reference

1 Hoult J, Renolds I, Charbonneau-Powis M, Weekes P, Briggs J (1983). Psychiatric hospital versus community treatment: the results of a randomised trial. *Australian and New Zealand Journal of Psychiatry* **17**: 160–7.

☼ Early intervention services

- The prognosis of schizophrenia has remained largely unchanged in spite of developments in medication and psychosocial interventions. Early intervention services in psychosis have been developed to improve the prognosis, although no-one would question that, as is the case for most medical conditions, the earliest intervention possible must be theoretically best to prevent deterioration in chronic conditions.
- Early intervention services in the UK are usually geared to the detection and treatment of established psychosis. Elsewhere attempts have been made to intervene in prodromal or prepsychotic states.
- To date the evidence for intervening in the so-called prodromal phase of psychoses or when there are considered to be other early warning signs of impending psychosis is unclear and, indeed, two-thirds of such individuals identified as possibly having prodromal signs may not in fact progress to psychosis and need intervention.
- So-called prodromal signs of schizophrenia include:
  - Social withdrawal
  - Sleep disturbance
  - Lack of concentration
  - Depression
  - Appetite disturbance
  - Mild suspiciousness
  - Ideas of reference
  - Odd beliefs
  - Perceptual distortion.
- The latter symptoms tend to be more indicative of the development of schizophrenia than the former.
- In retrospect there is often a clear deterioration in personality and social functioning, and falling away from developmental milestones in those developing schizophrenia. There is evidence of brain changes accompanying prodromal decline and predating the onset of positive psychotic symptoms.
- However, intervening prodromally risks falsely labelling and inappropriately treating individuals who will not develop psychosis with medication that has significant side-effects.
- Even the rare studies indicating the benefits of early intervention with high-risk prodromal populations, e.g. combining low-dose atypical antipsychotic medication and psychotherapy and/or specific psychological approaches, have been criticized on the basis that, on close examination, it is often found that some patients included in the studies often are noted to be already experiencing positive psychotic symptoms.

Reasons for early intervention

This rests on a number of hypotheses:

1. That the duration of untreated psychosis will affect the outcome, perhaps owing to such episodes of untreated psychosis being neurotoxic. However, such a relationship may be compounded by the fact that those with long periods of untreated psychosis are more likely to have an insidious onset with prominent negative symptoms and poor premorbid functioning, and thus come to psychiatric attention later. Clearly, reducing the length of untreated psychosis, even if the long-term prognosis is unaffected, may reduce the stress to patients and their families.

2. The critical period hypothesis, i.e. the first 3 years of schizophrenia have been considered to be the time of maximum deterioration in social functioning and a period where resistant positive psychotic symptoms emerge. The level of disability within such a period often predicts the long-term prognosis.

3. Early intervention may better meet the special needs of the then usually young patients, and avoid adversive and traumatic first experiences of psychiatric services, e.g. from severe side-effects of psychotropic medication and enforced hospitalization, which in turn may lead to a long-term adverse attitude to engaging with psychiatric services.

Currently, the duration of untreated psychosis is often long, between 1 and 2 years, and contact with and treatment from psychiatric services often commences after insight is lost.

The approaches of early intervention services

- These are as follows:
  - Early detection through education of the community, anti-stigma campaigns, and training of professionals.
  - In an acute phase of a first episode of psychosis, the emphasis is on multidisciplinary assessment.
  - A broader approach to detecting psychosis rather than on emphasis on the narrow diagnostic criteria of schizophrenia.
  - Initiating treatment in the community with as low a dose of atypical antipsychotics as possible.
  - Emphasis on therapeutic engagement.
- Following recovery there is emphasis on:
  - Ensuring compliance with antipsychotic medication.
  - Psychological treatment, particularly cognitive behavioural therapy, as an adjunct to medication.
  - Involving the user.
  - Psycho-educating carers.
  - Family intervention. There is an emphasis on partnership with the family, who remain the biggest source of support, or potential hindrance, to progress.
  - Emphasis on assisting the individual to self-monitor for the emergence of early warning signs of relapse and on other relapse prevention strategies.

Models of early intervention services

- These include:
  - Such an approach being incorporated into community mental health teams.
  - A stand-alone early intervention service.
  - A 'hub and spoke' model in which a central specialist service supports mainstream services to provide specialist input.
- There is evidence that early and assertive intervention in first episodes of psychosis may improve the outcome. The Early Psychosis Prevention and Intervention Centre (EPPIC) in Melbourne, Australia, has produced the best known evidence for better outcome, including in terms of quality of life and social functioning, lower requirements for antipsychotic medication, and shorter periods in hospital, together with evidence that such an approach is more cost-effective. Questions remain, however, about who should be targeted for such approaches, and what components of such early intervention services are, in fact, effective.
- Currently, individuals who come to psychiatric attention have often suffered from several years of untreated psychosis, lost their self-esteem, have a changed identity, and poor social functioning and aspirations.

Aims of early intervention service

- Include the following:
  - Reducing the duration of untreated psychosis.
  - Elimination of positive psychotic symptoms as they emerge.
  - Reduction of suicide rates, which are often highest during the early years of psychosis.
  - Reduction of relapse rates.
  - Reduction of incidence of post-traumatic stress disorder.
  - Specific psychological approaches.
- Positive psychotic symptoms do not always correlate with social dysfunction, and evidence from early intervention studies shows that psychological containment can be equivalent to medication when outcome is considered.
- There is also evidence from studies looking at adopted-away individuals who subsequently develop schizophrenia, that those in stable adoptive families show fewer symptoms than those in unstable adoptive family situations.

In conclusion, it is likely that there will be further development of such specialist modernization teams as described here, albeit within perhaps enhanced community mental health teams. Other groups that may be targeted might include those with personality disorder.

Mental health legislation relevant to emergencies in psychiatry

Mental Health Act 1983 (England and Wales) *294*
Definition of categories of mental disorder recognized in the Mental Health Act 1983 *296*
Orders under the Mental Health Act 1983 *301*
Mental Health Review Tribunals (MHRT) *301*
Mental Health Act Commission (MHAC) (Section 121) *302*
Court of Protection (Section 94) *302*
Patients' rights under Mental Health Act 1983 *303*
Consent to treatment *303*
Detention under the Mental Health Act on a general medical or surgical ward *304*
Changes to Mental Health Act 1983 introduced by Mental Health Act 2006 *305*
Mental Capacity Act 2005 *306*
Assessment of capacity under the Mental Capacity Act 2005 *306*
Provisions of Mental Capacity Act 2005 *306*
Mental Capacity Act 2005 *307*
Code of practice for Mental Capacity Act 2005 *308*

In the UK there are different legal systems for England and Wales, Scotland, and Northern Ireland, although they have developed in parallel.

UK mental health legislation covers more than the compulsory detention of patients, although it is this that is usually concentrated on in descriptions of the relevant Mental Health Act.

Mental Health Act 1983 (England and Wales)

In general, compulsory hospitalization depends not only on a diagnosis of mental disorder within the meaning of the Act in question, but also its necessity for the patient's health, safety, and/or for the protection of others.

Definition of categories of mental disorder recognized in the Mental Health Act 1983

Mental disorder

The Mental Health Act sets out (in Section 1) a broader definition of the term mental disorder, and then four specific categories within this. According to the Act, the term mental disorder means:
• Mental illness
• Arrested or incomplete development of mind
• Psychopathic disorder
• Any other disorder or disability of mind.
It excludes the following, which are, not grounds for detention in hospital under the Act, if *only*:
• Promiscuity/immoral conduct
• Sexual deviancy
• Dependence on alcohol or drugs.

Mental illness

Mental illness is undefined in the Mental Health Act 1983, but implies previous health and is taken to include psychosis, both functional and organic, and neurotic disorders, including anorexia or bulimia nervosa.

Arrested or incomplete development of mind

This includes:
• *Severe mental impairment*: a state of arrested or incomplete development of mind, which includes severe impairment of intelligence and social functioning, and is associated with abnormally aggressive or seriously irresponsible conduct on the part of the person concerned.
• *Mental impairment*: as above, but *'significant'* in place of 'severe'.
   There is no reference in the Act to IQ levels, only social performance. However, the degree of *mental retardation* (deficiency, subnormality, learning disability), i.e. intellectual deficit from birth or early age, is roughly *mild mental retardation* (IQ 50–70) in *mental impairment*, and *moderate to severe mental retardation* (IQ below 50) in *severe mental impairment* (i.e. *mental impairment* − mental retardation + abnormally aggressive or seriously irresponsible conduct).

Psychopathic disorder

This is a persistent disorder or disability of mind (whether or not including significant impairment of intelligence) which results in abnormally aggressive or seriously irresponsible conduct on the part of the person.
This is a legal diagnosis and can include the clinical diagnoses of psychopathy, antisocial or dissocial and, indeed, all personality disorders. One should look for general social malfunctioning, e.g. immaturity and difficulty in sustaining relationships and work, not just for antisocial behaviour.

Table 20.1 Civil treatment orders under Mental Health Act 1983

Civil treatment order under Mental Health Act 1983	Grounds	Application by	Medical recommendations	Maximum duration	Eligibility for appeal to Mental Health Review Tribunal
Section 2 Admission for assessment	Mental disorder	Nearest relative or approved social worker	Two doctors (one approved under Section 12)	28 days	Within 14 days
Section 3 Admission for treatment	Mental illness, psychopathic disorder, mental impairment, severe mental impairment. (If psychopathic disorder or mental impairment, treatment must be likely to alleviate or prevent deterioration)	Nearest relative or approved social worker	Two doctors (one approved under Section 12)	6 months	Within first 6 months, renewed, within second 6 months, then every year. Mandatory every 3 years
Section 4 Emergency admission for assessment	Mental disorder (urgent necessity)	Nearest relative or approved social worker	Any doctor	72 hours	
Section 5 (2) Urgent detention of voluntary inpatient	Danger to self or to others		Doctor in charge of patient's care	72 hours	

Table 20.1 (*Contd.*)

Civil treatment order under Mental Health Act 1983	Grounds	Application by	Medical recommendations	Maximum duration	Eligibility for appeal to Mental Health Review Tribunal
Section 5(4) Nurses holding power of voluntary inpatient	Mental disorder (danger to self, health, or others)	Registered mental nurse or registered nurse for mental handicap	None	6 hours	
Section 136 Admission by police	Mental disorder	Police officer	Allow patient in public place to be removed to 'place of safety'	72 hours	
Section 135	Mental disorder	Magistrates	Allows power of entry to home and removal of patient to place of safety	72 hours	

Table 20.2 Forensic treatment orders for mentally abnormal offenders

	Grounds	Made by	Medical recommendations	Maximum duration	Eligibility for appeal to Mental Health Review Tribunal
Section 35 Remand to hospital for report	Mental disorder	Magistrates or Crown Court	Any doctor	28 days. Renewable at 28-day intervals. Maximum12 weeks	
Section 36 Remand to hospital for treatment	Mental illness, severe mental impairment (not if charged with murder)	Crown Court	Two doctors (one approved under Section 12)	28 days. Renewable at 28-day intervals. Maximum 12 weeks	
Section 37 Hospital and guardianship months orders annually	Mental disorder. (If psychopathic disorder or mental impairment must be likely to alleviate or prevent deterioration.) Accused of, or convicted for, an imprisonable offence	Magistrates or Crown Court	Two doctors (one approved under Section 12)	6 months. Renewable for further 6 months, and then annually	During second 6 months. Then every year. Mandatory every 3 years
Section 41 Restriction order	Added to Section 37. To protect public from serious harm	Crown Court	Oral evidence from doctor	Usually without limit of time. Effect: leave, transfer, or discharge only with consent of Home Secretary	As Section 37
Section 38 Interim hospital order	Mental disorder. For trial of treatment	Magistrates or Crown Court	Two doctors (one approved under Section 12)	12 weeks. Renewable at 28-day intervals. Maximum 1 year	None

Table 20.2 (Contd.)

	Grounds	Made by	Medical recommendations	Maximum duration	Eligibility for appeal to Mental Health Review Tribunal
Section 47 Transfer of a sentenced prisoner to hospital	Mental disorder	Home Secretary	Two doctors (one approved under Section 12)	Until earliest date of release from sentence	Once in the first 6 months. Then once in the next 6 months. Thereafter, once a year.
Section 48 Urgent transfer to hospital of remand prisoner	Mental disorder	Home Secretary	Two doctors (one approved under Section 12)	Until date of trial	Once in the first 6 months. Then once in the next 6 months. Thereafter, once a year
Section 49 Restriction direction	Added to Section 47 or Section 48	Home Secretary	—	Until end of Section 47 and 48. Effect: leave, transfer, or discharge only with consent of Home Secretary	As for Section 47 and 48 to which applied

Orders under the Mental Health Act 1983

These are shown in Tables 20.1 and 20.2. These are also referred to as Sections, the numbers of which, in fact, refer to paragraph numbers in the Act. Knowledge of the use of such Sections relevant to emergency psychiatric situations is essential not only for psychiatrists but also GPs and casualty officers. Standard forms are available for application for each Section and are set out in a way that facilitates easy completion. Each order has a maximum duration, but most are reviewable.

Mental Health Review Tribunals (MHRT)

- Independent bodies consisting of doctor, lawyer, and lay person whose responsibility is to consider the justification for continued detention under the 1983 Mental Health Act.
- Chairman is a lawyer, and in the case of restricted patients, is usually a Judge.
- Patients are allowed legal aid to assist in representation, e.g. private psychiatric reports can be commissioned.
- Can order discharge or delayed discharge, and recommend (not order) transfer to another hospital or leave of absence or delayed discharge, e.g. in 1 month's time.
- Can also order discharge or conditional discharge (i.e. with conditions such as place of residence), or a deferred conditional discharge pending the conditions being met, of a Section 41 restricted patient.
- Can reclassify type of mental disorder.
- See eligibility for hearings in Tables 20.1 and 20.2.

Patients on a 72-h detention order have no MHRT rights, but can appeal against detention to hospital managers.

There are no MHRTs in Scotland, but there is a Mental Welfare Commission, which safeguards the rights of both voluntary and detained patients, and has the power to discharge patients.

Mental Health Act Commission (MHAC) (Section 121)

This is a special health authority, an independent body of about 100 part-time members (doctors, nurses, psychologists, social workers, lawyers, and lay people), appointed by the Secretary of State for Health.

• Provides approved doctors to give second opinions on consent to treatment.
• Receives, reviews, and scrutinizes detention documents and exercises a general protective function for all detained patients.
• Regularly visits psychiatric hospitals to interview detained patients and make sure their complaints are being properly handled. Visits special hospitals monthly and other psychiatric hospitals once or twice a year.
• Responsible for Code of Practice (Section 118) on detention, treatment of all psychiatric patients (informal or detained), and consent to treatment, etc. for the guidance of clinical and administrative staff in psychiatric hospitals and social workers.

Court of Protection (Section 94)

This is for the protection and management of the property of mentally disordered patients.

• Medical evidence that any form of mental disorder renders a person incapable of managing his property and affairs can be put to a judge in the special Court of Protection.
• If the judge is satisfied, he may then appoint a Receiver to act on behalf of the patient, keep his accounts, and manage his affairs.
• The receiver may be a relative, friend, solicitor, bank trustee or an official solicitor of the Supreme Court.
• The patient and his affairs may be checked from time to time by medical and legal visitors appointed by the Lord Chancellor.
• Medical visitors must have special knowledge and experience of mental disorder.
• Used especially for dementing patients, but also for those suffering from other mental disorders, such as mania and schizophrenia.

Patients' rights under Mental Health Act 1983

On admission, detained patients must be advised of their legal status, their rights to appeal to Mental Health Review Tribunals, their rights in respect of consent to treatment, those who have the authority to discharge them, and about the Mental Health Act Commission.

Correspondence to and from informal patients cannot be interfered with. Correspondence from detained patients in ordinary psychiatric hospitals can only be withheld if the person to whom the correspondence is addressed has asked for that to happen. Special hospitals such as Broadmoor Hospital can withhold correspondence to and from patients, except about staff and to solicitors and MPs or the sovereign. In the latter case, such correspondence can be sent free as it is to Royal Mail. Patients in any psychiatric hospital must be informed if their correspondence is withheld.

Informal patients have voting rights.

Health and social services have a duty to provide aftercare for detained patients when they leave hospital.

Consent to treatment

Consent to treatment should be informed and voluntary (implies mental illness, e.g. dementia, does not affect judgement). Provisions for treatment under the Mental Health Act 1983 are shown in Table 20.3.

Table 20.3 Consent to treatment under Mental Health Act 1983

Type of treatment	Informal	Detained
Urgent treatment **Section 57**	No consent	No consent
Irreversible, hazardous or non-established treatments, e.g. psychosurgery (e.g. leucotomy), hormone implants (for sex offenders), surgical operations (e.g. castration)	Consent and second opinion	Consent and second opinion
Section 58		
Psychiatric drugs, ECT	Consent	Consent or second opinion

1. For first 3 months of treatment a detained patient's consent is not required for Section 58 medicines, but is for ECT.

2. Patients can withdraw voluntary consent at any time.

❂ Detention under the Mental Health Act on a general medical or surgical ward

It is useful to be aware of the provisions of Section 5(2) for urgent detention of a voluntary inpatient, and Section 5(4), a nurse's holding of a voluntary inpatient. Section 5(2) can be used where a doctor thinks an assessment under the Mental Health Act ought to be undertaken with a view to detention under Section 2 (technically an assessment section for up to 28 days, but treatment can be undertaken during it) or Section 3 (a treatment section for up to 6 months) of the Mental Health Act 1983. It only applies to inpatients. Section 5(2) must be undertaken by the registered medical practitioner in charge of treatment (the consultant in charge of the patient's care or a deputy, e.g. an on-call doctor nominated by him). Section 5(2) cannot be used in accident and emergency departments or with outpatients. It does not allow treatment to be given in itself, although this can be done under Common Law or the Mental Capacity Act 2005. Section 5(2) lasts for 72 h and cannot be reapplied back to back at its expiry. The patient cannot be transferred to another ward as they are technically in a 'place of safety' unless the patient's life is at risk and there would be irreversible serious harm done.

In practice, additional security staff, or even police attendance, may be necessary when applying the provisions of Sections 5(2) or 5(4) to an uncooperative patient, and this should be considered. It is the medical or surgical team that is the responsible team and must complete the relevant sections if a patient is on a general hospital ward.

There are areas in the Section 5(2) form that require completion to indicate why informal treatment is no longer appropriate. Indications of this may include suspected mental illness, refusal to stay voluntarily in hospital, and risk to themselves or others.

As is the case for Mental Health Act 1983 Section application forms, accurate completion (including accurate spelling of the name!) of the legal paperwork is essential including the correct Trust and details of the patient.

Changes to Mental Health Act 1983 introduced by Mental Health Act 2006

1. *Single definition of mental disorder*
   - Any disorder or disability of the mind
   - Excludes learning disability unless associated with abnormally aggressive or seriously irresponsible conduct
   - Promiscuity, immoral conduct, and sexual deviancy no longer barred, but dependence on alcohol or drugs excluded.
2. *Treatability test replaced with test of available appropriate medical treatment with therapeutic purpose of improving patients condition or preventing deterioration.*
3. *Responsible clinicians*: designated by hospital and who may not be psychiatrists, take on role of Responsible Medical Officer (RMO) but must be *approved clinicians* according to Secretary of State.
   - *Approved mental health professionals* (AMHP) replace approved social workers and may not be social workers, but still to be approved by local Social Services Authority.
4. *Community treatment order (CTO)*
   - Supervised community treatment (SCT) of a 'community patient' granted by responsible clinician but agreed by AMHP
   - Power to recall to hospital if risk of harm to patient or others or conditions breached.
   - Initially for 6 months, but renewable for a further 6 months and then a year, etc
   - Section 25A goes.
5. *Nearest relative*
   - To include 'civil partners'.
   - Power of patients to apply to court to specify person.
6. *Forensic psychiatric cases*
   - Requirement for agreement between clinicians as to particular type of mental disorder under Section 37 removed.
   - Courts can no longer limit length of Section 41 Restriction Order
7. *Mental health review tribunals*
   - Powers extended to community treatment orders.
   - 6-month maximum for referral by hospital managers in absence of application by patient
8. *Draft code of practice*
   - Guidance over Bournewood gap patients.
   - New guidance for long-term seclusion.

Mental Capacity Act 2005

The Mental Capacity Act 2005 came into effect partially in April 2007 and fully from October 2007. Prior to the Mental Capacity Act 2005, patients lacking capacity could be treated under Common Law, under which a doctor must treat an incapable patient in their best interests as the doctor has a 'duty of care' (doctrine of necessity).

The Mental Capacity Act has five main principles:

- The person must be assumed to have capacity unless it is established that he lacks capacity.
- An individual should not be regarded as unable to make a decision unless all practical steps to help him do so have been undertaken without success.
- An individual is not to be treated as unable to make a decision merely because he makes an unwise decision.
- Any action or decision made under the Act for, or on behalf of, an individual who lacks capacity must be done in his best interests.
- Regard must be taken before an act is done or a decision made under the Act as to whether the purpose can be effectively achieved in a less restrictive way in terms of the patient's rights and freedom of action.

Assessment of capacity under the Mental Capacity Act 2005

This is a two-stage process:

1. Is there impairment or disturbance in the functioning of the person's mind or brain?
2. If there is, does this make the person unable to make a particular decision?

The Act states that the question should be decided on a balance of probabilities. The following are considered central to the assessment:

- Understanding information relevant to the decision.
- Retaining that information.
- Ability to use or weigh up that information as part of the process of making the decision.
- Ability to communicate the decision, which can include means other than talking such as sign language or writing.

Provisions of Mental Capacity Act 2005

The Mental Capacity Act sets out the legal requirements for making decisions on behalf of patients who lack capacity.

- It enables patients to plan ahead for a time when they lack capacity.
- It provides protection both for the incompetent patient and those who have to make decisions about their care.

Mental Capacity Act 2005

Designated decision makers for those who lack capacity

Lasting Powers of Attorney (LPAs)
- Like the pre-existing Enduring Power of Attorney (EPA) but can make health and welfare decisions on behalf of the individual.

Court-appointed deputies
- Replaces Receivership in the Court of Protection.
- Can make decisions on welfare, healthcare, and financial matters, but will not be able to refuse consent to life-sustaining treatment.

Two new public bodies
- A new Court of Protection
- A new Public Guardian
  - Will register LPAs and deputies
  - Supervise deputies
  - Be scrutinized by a Public Guardian Board

Three provisions to protect vulnerable people
- Independent Mental Capacity Advocate (IMCA).
- Advance decisions to refuse treatment, including, if expressly stated, 'even if life is at risk'.
- New criminal offence of ill treatment or neglect of person who lacks capacity.

Code of practice for Mental Capacity Act 2005

Key points in this include:

1. Capacity should be assessed each time there is a separate decision to be taken, but there may be patients whose absence of capacity remains constant. Each assessment of capacity should be recorded.
2. *Best interests*: clinicians and staff 'must be able to point to objective reasons to demonstrate why they believe they are acting in the person's best interest'.
3. *Restraint*: this does not mean physical restraint alone, but can refer to a restriction in liberty of movement, e.g. a secure lock on a door leading to a busy main road. It must be reasonable and proportionate to circumstances, e.g. it would be inappropriate to lock someone in a bedroom continuously owing to a tendency to wander out into the road.

The Mental Capacity Act was amended by the Mental Health Act 2006 to introduce 'Detained Resident' status to plug the Bournewood gap of patients who lack capacity and remain in hospitals or care homes informally as regards the Mental Health Act 1983.

Applications are to be made to Primary Care Trusts (PCT) for hospitals and Local Authority for care homes, except in Wales, where they are to be made to the National Assembly.

Protective care orders for detained residents

- Age 18 or over
- Mental disorder as defined in MHA, plus learning disability alone included
- Lack of mental capacity to decide whether should be in hospital or care home for treatment
- 'Best interests' requirement. Detention should be proportionate
- Eligible even if subject to Mental Health Act
- 'No refusals' requirement, e.g. resulting from a valid Advance Directive or LPA
- IMCAs will support and represent detained residents

Impact

- In 2004–5 42 900 formal Mental Health Act 1983 assessments in England and Wales led to 14 700 detentions in England and 545 in Wales
- Estimate for Mental Capacity Act, 5000 subject to Bournewood assessment and 1250 deprived of liberty.
  However, in the UK:
- 210 000 have severe/profound learning disability
- 1.2 million have mild to moderate learning disability
- 700 000 have dementia
- 120 000 have severe brain injury.

Difficult patients and difficult situations

Psychodynamic aspects of the management of psychiatric
    emergencies *310*
Managing difficult patients *312*
Understanding the psychodynamics of being mentally
    disordered *314*
Particular situations of difficulty *316*

⊙ Psychodynamic aspects of the management of psychiatric emergencies

Transference
- Patients project onto staff strong emotions from the past, e.g. professionals are seen as authority figure representing, perhaps, the patients' abusive parents. Do not take anger personally. With aggressive personalities, young therapists may do better than older parental figures.

Countertransference
- Behaviour including violence or offence, e.g. paedophilia, produces strong emotions in staff who can feel shocked or overwhelmed, leading to negative countertransference feelings of dislike. This can lead on to overestimation of risk and inappropriate precipitate action to cover self and displace responsibility onto others, e.g. calling police, or an attempt to rescue dangerous untreatable people and denying what one does not want to hear. There is a need to maintain judgement. A feeling of fear can be a good warning sign if you understand your own feelings.

Splitting
- Patient sees current professional or part of a multidisciplinary team as good and all other professionals as having been bad, but idealization is often followed by denigration.

Projective identification
- Makes you feel as they do, e.g. frightened, anxious. Even if patients are angry, remember they usually feel worse than you.

Staffs' role in precipitating violence
- While usually unintended, staff often avoid consideration of their role or blame self and feel responsible (a normal human psychological defence mechanism as an alternative to an unpredictable and dangerous world).

Psychodynamic formulation of violence
- Predisposition
  - Owing to childhood traumas, making it difficult to tolerate painful feelings.
- Precipitants
  - Current circumstances seen as repetition of trauma leading to projection onto staff of negative feelings towards, e.g. previously abusive parents, and acting out.
  - Perpetuating factors: the more fragile the psychological defences, the more violence.

It is better to concentrate on the 'here and now' rather than family and early background factors.
- Other psychodynamic issues
  - Identification with aggressor e.g. client becomes angry if challenged that parents may have been abusive to them.
- Repetition—compulsion. Leads to self-defeating behaviour.
- Displaced aggressiveness towards e.g. staff but directed towards parents. 'Unfinished business'—is the victim the actual individual with whom the client is angry. This also leads to formal complaints.
- Disruption of therapeutic alliance, e.g. staff leave aggravates clients' fear of rejection.
- Seeking physical security to contain emotional insecurity, e.g. client becomes violent to be removed from community where they are unable to cope and to obtain the security of detention or imprisonment. Aim to contain such feelings of emotional insecurity.
- Seeking of instant cure, e.g. tablets.
- Bottomless pit: staff can never meet clients' needs after the client discovers the first person in their life in whom they can confide. Patient burden transferred to staff.
- Murderous thoughts can be normal. Acting on them is not.
- Fear of madness and losing control.
- Amnesia for violence: this may be due to hysterical denial, substance abuse or reduced memory registration due to overarousal (comparable to exam phobia), not merely lying.
- Patients with personality disorder often ambivalent and hostile about seeking and need for treatment.
- Under stress, people often become either more inhibited or more generally dominating and aggressive.
- Staff may not always be able to help and it can be useful to accept all you can do is what you can do.

Reference

1 Treasaden IH (2003). Assessment of violence in medium secure units. In: Doctor R (ed.) *Dangerous Patients. A psychodynamic approach to risk assessment and risk management.* Karnac: London.

Managing difficult patients

It is important to appreciate that acutely psychotic patients may hold catastrophic cognitions, including anxiogenic cognitions such as a fear of being locked up or of being untreatable or of progressively deteriorating, and of depressogenic cognitions of hopelessness, despair, and suicidal ideation. The content of delusions, hallucinations, and thought disorder may indicate emotionally pertinent themes important to the patient.

The paranoid patient

A professional should adopt a non-threatening body position, avoiding prolonged eye contact and invasion of body space. Talking indirectly in the third person may be preferential to doing so in the second person, i.e. 'you …'. Try to be empathic, non-judgemental, and have a reciprocal emotional tone. Do not challenge or confront delusional beliefs in emergency situations. This may entrench and worsen such delusions and be met with anger (this is in contrast to non-urgent situations, in which a cognitive behavioural therapy approach may be adopted to counter delusions by peripheral and Socratic questioning to modify beliefs).

Antisocial personality

Interviews with such patients are often facilitated if they are allowed to communicate freely their opinions and views. If they threaten antisocial behaviour as a result of their problems, try to offer reality-orientated alternatives. Avoid provocation. To tell an antisocial personality, who may be threatening self-harm or harm to others, that he has a condition that psychiatrists cannot help is likely to provoke the individual to act on such threats. Short-term courses of medication or admission to hospital may allow them to cool off, even if such treatment in the long-term is of less certain benefit. To engage antisocial patients one may need to accept late arrival for appointments or unannounced presentation. Be flexible within considered limits beyond which you will not go. Such patients often do better with younger therapists than older, who represent authority figures to them. They should be advised that they are legally responsible for their actions, and that this is not affected even if prescribed symptomatic psychotropic medication to assist them.

Borderline and histrionic personalities

Such individuals may present in an overemotional and overdramatic fashion and be prone to repetitive self-harm and overdoses of medication. Uncritical acceptance and an attempt at demonstrating empathic understanding is required to try and reinforce their usually low self-esteem and their self-cognition that they have 'failed again' when they present to psychiatric services. Their behaviour may appear attention-seeking, but this should elicit an attempt to try and determine what the patients themselves want to happen. Such patients need to be encouraged to accept responsibility for their actions.

Acute stress reactions

In such cases it is important to allow the patient time to ventilate their feelings.

✪ The manipulative patient

Some argue that one should never use the term 'manipulative' as it is pejorative and leads to a lack of clinical consideration of what underlies such behaviour, and rejection of the patient. Manipulativeness implies selfishness and maladaptive behaviour, but in general such behaviour always reflects genuine problems of the individual concerned. Common examples of behaviour that are regarded as manipulative include inappropriate and unrealistic demands, for instance, for hospital admission, a demand to be seen only by particular doctors, and out-of-hours presentations. Behind such demands are threats of behavioural sequelae, such as self-harm, violence, complaints or passive resistance.

The guiding principle is that clinicians should only respond appropriately and objectively to the clinical condition, not to such demands.

The practice of 'blacklisting' particular patients from admission is not to be recommended, as it does not allow for a change in clinical picture. While admission to hospital reinforces negative behaviour, a patient can always raise the stakes beyond which medical staff will not go, e.g. by increasing self-harm. While agreeing to an out-of-hours admission may result in a patient's responsible multidisciplinary team being critical, one should not feel you have lost and the patient has won as, in such a situation out-of-hours, even the patient's usual professionals would probably have had to respond in the same way. Always consult colleagues in such difficult decisions.

⑦ Understanding the psychodynamics of being mentally disordered

In all mentally disordered patients, but particularly when the illness is psychotic[1], be aware of the following:
1. Oversensitivity.
2. Dependency and increased egocentricity:a patient may be particularly sensitive to a professional who fails to keep an appointment.
3. Potential artificial nature of a psychotherapeutic approach:almost everyone has some elements of concern in their life regarding feelings of inadequacy, fear of being unable to form close relationships, and about their sexuality. Rather than indicating to a patient that if he leaves therapy, it is resistance, or that if he likes the therapist, it is transference, one needs to look at the individual patient's motives.
4. Failure to take patients seriously: studies show reduced eye contact between professionals and patients compared to normal social interactions.
5. Lack of information: a patient may particularly worry about the results of investigations if these are not fed back to him.
6. Boredom: psychiatric disorder may result in feeling too ill to concentrate.

7. Stigma: psychiatric patients often feel permanently different and affected. One should attempt to normalize their difficulties and point out that all individuals have their 'breaking point'. Psychiatric terminology may aggravate this; rather than call a patient paranoid, use terms such as insecure or suspicious.

8. Denial of illness: avoid overzealous challenging of denial. Gently present alternative explanations to those of the patient. Respect patients' points of view.

9. Terror: this may be countered by reassurance and often by the professional's mere presence. One may need to be guided by the patient as to whether they are left alone, subject to safety considerations.

10. Demoralization: professionals should be positive and hopeful, and enquire into the specific origins of demoralization rather than view it as part of the psychiatric disorder. Education and guidance may need to be given about negative symptoms to facilitate a sense of mastery by the patient of his condition and to counter low drive.

Reference

1 Weiden P, Havens L (1994). Psychotherapeutic management techniques in the treatment of outpatients with schizophrenia. *Hospital and Community Psychiatrist* **45**: 549–5.

Particular situations of difficulty

Demands for medication or hospital admission

This may be an appropriate demand in both cases if an individual is acutely mentally unwell or, in the case of demanding medication alone, has run out of their medication, but otherwise it is inappropriate and one may need to set limits. However, beware of the risk of provoking a patient to raise the stakes by merely dismissing such demands as unreasonable, e.g. if a patient is threatening to harm him or herself if you do not meet their demands. If it appears that the patient is not immediately suicidal at present, this may allow time for alternative supervision or management plans to be put in place. Short-term additional medication or hospital admission may allow an individual to cool off and not act out or self-harm, even if it will not affect the long-term course of the condition, e.g. personality disorder.

Demanding relatives

This may reflect the guilt and anxiety of the relatives themselves about the patient's condition and care. However, relatives are better medically, including psychiatrically, informed and more willing to challenge those in authority than was the case in the past. Remember, that while relatives can provide important third party information about a patient and his condition, in normal circumstances a patient's consent is required before they can be approached to this end. Also, remember relatives remain the main support in the community for most patients.

Threatening suicide by telephone calls

The advice in this difficult situation is usually to try and keep the patient talking and allow him to ventilate his or her feelings. An attempt should be made to identify the name and current location of the patient, and encourage them to attend hospital. If they refuse, emergency services can be contacted and the police may have the capacity to trace the individual. However, in general, such individuals tend to be similar to those who contact the Samaritans and who are at risk of deliberate self-harm rather than those with overwhelming suicidal intent.

Patients acting against medical advice, including taking their own discharge from hospital

It is assumed, unless contested, that every adult has the right and the capacity (legal concept) (competence) to decide whether or not he or she will accept medical treatment, even if refusal risks permanent injury to health or premature death.

A patient can therefore refuse treatment if there is no impairment of their capacity and they do not suffer from mental disorder of a nature or degree allowing compulsory treatment under the relevant Mental Health Act. Lack of capacity is not equivalent to detainability under the Mental Health Act 1983. Where it is uncertain if a patient lacks capacity, the advice is to act first and dispute later.

Some common examples follow.

A patient who has taken an overdose of medication wishes to take their discharge from an accident and emergency department against medical advice

Theoretically, if the patient has the capacity, they are entitled to do so. However, medical defence associations emphasize that self-harm or overdoses of medication are suggestive of mental disorder and, on this basis, if the clinician is in doubt, detention under the Mental Health Act is defendable. Remember that the definition of mental disorder in the Mental Health Act is a legal definition equivalent to a lay person's and not equivalent to an ICD-10 or DSM-IV diagnosis.

Alcohol dependency

While dependence on alcohol alone is excluded from the definition of mental disorder required for detention under the Mental Health Act, detention may be justifiable on the grounds of associated depression, e.g. if it is considered that the individual is at risk to himself.

Alcohol intoxication

This may result in impaired capacity, and, as such, urgent treatment can be undertaken on the basis of a Common Law duty (justification of necessity) to act in the best possible interests of the patient.

An informal inpatient in a psychiatric unit wanting to take their discharge following admission

This is not an uncommon situation. Some individuals accept admission only to find the facilities unsatisfactory and the disturbed behaviour of other patients stressful. The default position is that a reassessment of the case is required at the time the patient asks for his discharge, following which the risks of discharge from hospital may be weighed up and, if necessary, formal detention under the Mental Health Act undertaken.

Decisions to involve police following violence or other serious offences on psychiatric inpatient units

- The majority of violence, for instance to nursing staff or other patients, never results in criminal charges.
- Serious violence, e.g. homicide, grievous bodily herm, is a matter for police involvement as it is a matter of public interest.
- Current zero tolerance policy towards violence to staff by patients is increasingly leading to police involvement. The onus should be on the hospital, not the victim, to press charges.
- Police involvement at least allows for independent investigation and documentation of incidents.
- Chances of conviction are often slight when it is one mentally disordered patient's allegation about another mentally disordered patient, in absence of other evidence, e.g. allegations of sexual assault or rape by one patient of another where the alleged perpetrator claims consent was given.
- Charging an inpatient with an offence may be unprofitable if the patient is clearly going to require ongoing inpatient treatment in the same facility.

- However, police involvement may reinforce to a patient the unacceptability of his or her behaviour, especially when it does not arise directly from the individual's mental illness
- Be aware that removal by police of an inpatient will not remove the patient's psychiatric difficulties, which are likely to lead to presentation to services again. Even if police remove an inpatient from a psychiatric inpatient unit and that patient is convicted of threats or assault, the likely time in custody will be short.

Lack of inpatient beds to admit patients

It is, of course, part of every doctor's task to manage the finite resources available to him or her. However, the legal advice is that if you cannot do your job properly, you should not attempt to do it at all.

Problems may arise when a formal mental health assessment is undertaken, a patient is deemed detainable under the relevant Mental Health Act, but no bed is available at the responsible catchment area psychiatric unit. The advice then is for the doctor to proceed and complete the formal application to the Hospital Managers for admission. It is then for the hospital authorities to find a bed, if necessary elsewhere, including in the private sector.

Emergencies in forensic psychiatry

Police and court liaison 320
Psychiatric expert evidence for court 324
Problem areas in police/court liasion and reporting 326
Prison psychiatry 328

Forensic psychiatrists assess and treat mentally abnormal offenders and are based in medium secure units, Special Hospitals, and prisons

Forensic psychiatrists may also be asked to provide advice on the management of, and treatment of, aggressive and other severely behaviourally disturbed patients who may not have technically offended.

Most general psychiatrists will, however, see a number of patients who offend each year

A forensic psychiatric assessment should include:

- Full history and mental state examination of the patient, including of fantasies and impulses to offend. In sexual offenders are such impulses egosyntonic or egodystonic?
- Objective account of offence, e.g. from arresting police officer or, in more serious cases before the Crown Court, from statements (depositions) of witnesses
- An objective account of past offences, if any. You can obtain a list of previous convictions from the probation service, court or solicitors
- Additional information-gathering, including interviews with informants such as relatives, and reading social enquiry reports prepared by probation officers
- Review of previous psychiatric records and reports, e.g. to ascertain relationship of mental disorder to previous behaviour and response to psychiatric treatment and need for security. Some individuals may continue to be violent and/or offend even after their mental illness is controlled.

Following an offence, an individual may be:

- Detained under a civil section of the Mental Health Act
- Cautioned by the police, which has to be accepted by the offender
- Charged
- If charged, an individual may be remanded on bail or in custody until the trial in court.

① Police and court liaison

Terminology
Diversion or early diversion
- Transfer to healthcare system of a mentally disordered individual in police custody or at first court hearing.

Diversion, or police or court diversion, schemes
- Specific psychiatric services are provided to the police and/or courts, usually to the Magistrates Court where 98% of offenders are tried. However, it is unlikely that serious offenders, e.g. those charged with murder, will be suitable for such diversion.

Psychiatric issues relevant to police and court liaison
- Evidence of mental disorder
- Need for outpatient or inpatient psychiatric treatment
- Urgency if inpatient psychiatric treatment required
- Nature of alleged offence and risk to others
- Fitness to remain in police custody

- Fitness to be interviewed by police
- Fitness to plead if is to appear in court.

Note should be taken of the following points:

- Remember, the technical legal offence may not reflect the actual risk. For example, arson may be of a waste paper bin in front of others on a busy hospital ward or committed with intent to endanger the lives of others in a tower block. Similarly, possession of an offensive weapon may have been with a view to seriously harming others.
- Offending is not a characteristic symptom of any mental disorder.
- Offence = offender × victim × situation.

☼ Fitness to remain in police custody

- No legal definition
- An individual may be unfit to remain in police custody due to physical illness or psychiatric disorder
- Serious and immediate risk to an individual's health will usually make the individual unfit to remain in police custody. Detention under a civil section of the Mental Health Act may then be indicated.

☼ Fitness to be interviewed by police

- No legal definition
- Individuals should be able to understand the police caution after it has been explained
- Full orientation to time, place, and person is required
- Fitness may be questioned if an individual is likely to give answers due to their mental disorder that may be wrongly interpreted by the Court
- If an individual is fit to be interviewed but has a history of mental disorder, then an appropriate adult should be present. Such individuals can be provided by appropriate adult schemes.

① Fitness to plead

This refers to the time of the trial and not the alleged offence.

An individual who is fit to plead must be able to do the following:

- Instruct counsel
- Appreciate the significance of pleading, i.e. to note the difference between saying guilty and not guilty
- Challenge a juror
- Examine a witness
- Understand and follow the evidence of Court procedure.

NB. The defendant does not have to be fit to give evidence himself. In England and Wales, under the Domestic Violence, Crime and Victims Act 2004, a Judge will first determine fitness to plead, then a trial of facts follows. A range of disposals, including Hospital Order, Supervision Order and Absolute Discharge, are available by way of sentence.

① False confessions[1]

Three types have been described.

1. Voluntary: for instance, due to depression or morbid guilt.
2. Coerced–compliant: owing to being pressurized during interrogation. Such false confessions are often retracted after interrogation.
3. Coerced–internalized: the individual becomes confused by interrogation and comes to believe false story. Particularly seen in learning disability.

In cases of possible suggestibility and false confessions:

- Assess intellectual level
- Gudjonnson suggestibility scale.

Reference

1 Gudjonnson GH (1993). *The psychology of Interrogations, Confessions and Testimony.* Chichester: Lodey.

① Psychiatric expert evidence for court

The following issues, with particular relevance to the legal position in England and Wales, are likely to have to be subsequently addressed in the opinion of a court report or in oral evidence to court:
1. Fitness to plead.
2. Mental responsibility.
   a. Not guilt by reason of insanity ('special verdict') (insanity defence) (McNaughton Rules). This refers to the time of the offence. Owing to disease of mind, either (i) the individual did not know the nature or quality of his act (physical nature of the act), or (ii) did not know what he was doing was wrong (forbidden by law). (iii) If an individual held delusional false beliefs, then his actions should be judged by their relationship to the delusion, e.g. if an individual is deluded that his life was immediately threatened, then he would be justified in striking out but not otherwise, e.g. if merely deluded that others were against him.
      Results in discretionary sentencing, including detention in hospital.
   b. Diminished responsibility This is a defence against the charge of murder alone.
      The individual has to show that, at the time he killed, he was suffering from 'such abnormality of mind … as substantially impaired his mental responsibility for his acts'.
      The effect of such a successful plea is to reduce the charge from murder, which carries a statutory mandatory sentence of life imprisonment, to manslaughter, where the court has the power of discretionary sentencing.
3. Nature of mental disorder, i.e. in England and Wales, mental illness, mental impairment, or psychopathic disorder under the Mental Health Act 1983.
4. Is the patient treatable?
5. Have arrangements been made for such treatment?
   For example, a Community Rehabilitation Order with a condition of outpatient psychiatric treatment or inpatient psychiatric treatment under Section 37 of the Mental Health Act 1983.
6. Is the patient dangerous?
   This may lead the Court to add a Restriction Order to the Hospital Order. In England and Wales this is under Section 41 of the Mental Health Act 1983 'to protect the public from serious harm', following which discharge, transfer or leave requires Home Office authorization, although a Mental Health Review Tribunal can order absolute discharge or conditional discharge with conditions, such as a specified place of residence such as a hostel, and compliance with statutory psychiatric and social worker supervision, or a deferred conditional discharge until such conditions are met.
   The degree of risk may mean that any inpatient treatment ought to be conducted under conditions of security, such as in a medium secure unit or a maximum secure Special Hospital such as Broadmoor, Ramp-

ton or Ashworth hospitals in England or Carstairs State Hospital in Scotland. Emergency admissions to medium secure units and Special Hospitals are not usually available. Special hospital admission depends on written referral with emphasis on details of actual incidents indicative of risk to others and absconding risk, and the potential receiving special hospital's assessment of the case itself.

Medium secure units are for those with mental disorder whose disruptive and/or dangerous behaviour requires psychiatric treatment in conditions of more security than ordinary hospital, including low secure locked psychiatric intensive care units, but less than Special Hospitals.

Special Hospitals are for the treatment of mental disorder in individuals requiring special (maximum) security (in fact, equivalent to a Category B prison) on account of their violent, dangerous or criminal propensities, i.e. immediate danger to the public if they were to abscond, and the fact that they cannot safely be managed in a medium secure unit.

7. Suggestions for non-psychiatric management, e.g. a Community Rehabilitation Order, a supervised hostel or care home.

① Problem areas in police/court liaison and reporting

If an individual is pleading not guilty or is undecided upon his plea but you think the individual was mentally ill at the time of the offence, say, e.g. 'for the time of the offence, Mr X showed symptoms of mental illness such as ...'. This avoids having to comment on likely guilt before a plea is entered.

Explaining the relationship of mental illness to offending

An offence may have arisen directly from paranoid or passivity delusions due to mental illness or indirectly owing to a deterioration in personality and social functioning, for instance in schizophrenia. There may be no relationship between the offence and mental disorder. The offence and legal consequences may precipitate a mental illness, e.g. depression.

Personality disorder

If you do not think that an individual's personality difficulties are amenable to specific inpatient psychiatric treatment, then say so and add, 'in the absence of mental illness and mental impairment I do not consider him detainable under the Mental Health Act 1983'.

Remember that, in England and Wales, the legal category of psychopathic disorder encompasses all clinical types of personality disorder but, for detention, the treatment offered must have the prospect of benefit.

Psychiatric and psychological treatment can be offered after the law has taken its course when the individual is free to take it up, or as a condition of a Community Rehabilitation (previously Probation) Order.

Substance misuse

In general it may be best to allow the law to take its course and only offer treatment/help on a voluntary basis when the individual is free to take this up, except where specific drug rehabilitation residential placements are recommended as a condition of, for instance, a Community Rehabilitation Order, to which, however, the patient must agree. In general, the advice is usually that the individual must stop abusing alcohol or drugs, that this is something the individual must primarily decide to do, although the ability or will of the individual to do so may be in doubt, but the individual may additionally be helped by services in doing so.

Problem of individuals citing hearing a 'voice' telling them to commit an offence where a mental illness is not suspected

Note the absence of other characteristic symptoms of severe mental illness, such as schizophrenia. Such isolated voices may reflect only pseudohallucinations which are usually perceived as in the mind rather than external space, occurring in individuals with severe personality disorder under stress, or may be due to substance abuse.

History of mild head injury or mild learning disability

Such a history does not necessarily imply that the condition is of a degree that would adversely affect the individual's ability to otherwise normally sustain himself adequately in the community and be responsible for their acts. Frequent problems occur in those of borderline learning disability who are not suitable for learning disability services, although the courts and social services look to the medical profession to manage such individuals in spite of the 'normal' intelligence level and that their offending is usually due to personality difficulties.

ⓘ Prison psychiatry

Psychiatrists may be requested to assess prisoners to:
- Provide court reports
- Provide assessments on management and advice, including for sentenced prisoners, at the request of Prison Medical Officers
- For statutory purposes, such as preparing reports for the Parole Board.

To visit a prisoner, arrangements will need to be made with the Healthcare Wing of the prison. Psychiatrists may need security clearance. Assessments will have to fit in with prison routine, which only allows for 2–3 h in the morning or the afternoon to see a patient, and the psychiatrist will usually need to wait for prison staff escorts upon arrival.

Issues relevant to psychiatric care in prison include the following:
- Prevention, i.e. of offending and imprisonment, by psychiatric care in the community.
- Police station/court diversion schemes.
- Screening should be undertaken on reception of inmates to prison (three-quarters of psychiatric cases may be missed owing to inadequate screening).
- Measures to counter suicide risk (highest in the first 2 months, especially among the young on remand who are not necessarily formally mentally ill).
- Return to psychiatric hospital care under the relevant Mental Health Act while on remand, by means of court sentence or during custodial sentence.
- Substance misuse/detox services. Abstinence may result in a medical emergency due to withdrawal. Also, there are high mortality rates in cases of substance misuse upon release from prison owing to loss of tolerance.
- Sex Offender Treatment Programmes (SOTP).
- Special therapeutic community units for sentenced prisoners with personality disorder, e.g. HMP Grendon in England.
- Dangerous severe personality disorder (DSPD) Units at HMP Whitmoor and HMP Franklin.

NB. The Mental Health Act does not apply in prison, but medical treatment can be administered in good faith under Common Law in prison where there is lack of capacity to consent and in the best interests of the individual, e.g. to prevent immediate serious risk to others or self.

The aim is that healthcare in prison should be equivalent to NHS care outside, with 24-h psychiatric care/inreach for remanded and sentenced prisoners, on both medical wings and ordinary locations, provided by local general or forensic mental health services.

☺ Suicide risk in prison

This is nine times higher than in the community and highest in the first 2 months in custody. Formal mental illness may be absent.

At-risk groups include:
- Those on remand
- Young

- Those with a history of substance misuse
- Those with a history of violent offences

Other factors, such as anxiety about the consequences of future court hearings, bullying, isolation, and poor conditions in prison may also be relevant.

Assessment is often compounded by the limited information available in prison. Attempts should be made to gather background history, including from psychiatric services previously involved in the care of an individual.

Prediction remains difficult. Suicide remains the most common cause of death in prisons and is most commonly by hanging.

NB. While the prevalence of mental disorder in prison populations is high, with perhaps the majority suffering from mental disorder, albeit mainly personality disorder and/or substance misuse, the criterion for transfer to hospital under the Mental Health Act is that an individual requires detention for inpatient psychiatric treatment, not merely that the individual might benefit from psychiatric or psychological help, including in prison.

A useful guide when assessing offenders as regards to their need for psychiatric treatment is to ignore the offence and assess the need for treatment as if one were seeing them as a new outpatient case.

⑦ Coroners' Courts

- The Court most often attended by the medical profession
- Coroners should be called Sir when being addressed
- The verdict must not be framed in a way to determine civil liability
- Coroners' Courts are understanding of the difficulties of managing outpatients prone to self-harm under stress.

⑦ Psychiatric opinions in Civil Law (civil capacity)

Burden of proof is on the balance of probabilities, in contrast to criminal courts where it is beyond reasonable doubt.

Civil law refers to citizens' rights and civil wrongs, and involves one individual against another as regards matters defined by Parliament and the courts as civil, including negligence and the administration of the Mental Health Act. This is in contrast to criminal law, where it is the State that initiates proceedings on behalf of society.

Civil law issues that may be relevant to emergency situations in psychiatry include the following:

Issues of mental fitness

- Testamentary capacity (ability to make a valid will)
- Treatment refusal.

Issues of psychiatric damage

- Legal term is 'nervous shock'
- The vulnerability of the complainant is not relevant, i.e. an 'eggshell skull' is no defence
- For psychiatric damage an individual must have a psychiatric illness
- Psychiatric damage can be:
  - Secondary to physical sequelae, e.g. after loss of a limb
  - Primary: psychological
  - Psychological but secondary, e.g. witnessing the fate of another

Damages are to compensate not punish, hence will be greater for brain damage than death.

Psychiatric negligence

- There are three elements:
  - A duty of care to a 'neighbour'
  - Breach of duty of care, includes technical advice errors
  - Damage to other party results, i.e. foreseeable and would not have happened anyway
- The onus of proof is on the plaintiff to prove breach of duty of care caused damage
- Common causes of psychiatric negligence, in order of frequency:
  - *Suicide or attempted suicide (50%)*
    - Failure of assessment or management, including good operational suicide policies, documentation of suicide risk and management plan, and the informing of all relevant staff, including observing nursing staff.
  - *Negligent use of drugs (30%)*
    - Particularly drug toxicity, especially lithium. This may involve the wrong drug being prescribed, the patient not being properly monitored or not being properly warned, or no proper consent procedure.
    - For lithium there may be:
      - Delays in the laboratory telling the doctor the result
      - Failure to check thyroid or renal functioning
      - Failure to monitor blood levels
      - Most caused by use of diuretics
      - Failure to diagnose organic disorders.
  - *Other causes include*
    - Homicide by patient
    - Sexual misconduct of doctor
    - Breach of confidentiality
    - Lack of supervision (advice, instruction, monitoring and control), e.g. by consultant of trainee
    - Cases are scrutinized to see if 'reasonable care' compared to professional peers was present
    - An error of judgement or mistake becomes negligent if the individual did not exercise reasonable care
    - Cases arise from a bad outcome plus bad feelings, guilt, rage, grief or surprise.

Index

A

abdominal symptoms 186–7
Abortion Act 1967 244–5
Absolute Discharge 321
abuse, violence and disaster, victims of 87
adjustment disorder 106
child abduction 89
childhood sexual abuse, consequences for adult functioning of 89
elder abuse 92
erotomania (de Clérambault's) 95
morbid jealousy (Othello syndrome) 93
non-accidental injury of children 88
post-traumatic stress disorder 100–4
rape and sexual assault of men 98–9
rape and sexual assault of women 96–7
spouse abuse 90–1
stalking 95
stress reaction, acute 106
accident and emergency departments 183–9
discharge from 271
medically unexplained symptoms 188
Munchausen syndrome (hospital addiction syndrome) 186–7
old-age psychiatry 266
accidents 140
activated charcoal 31
Acuphase 76
acute stress reactions 312
Addisonian crisis 56
adjustment disorder 106
adolescents see children and adolescents
adoption psychosis 237
adult advanced cardiac arrest life support algorithm 35
advance decisions to refuse treatment 306
aggression and violence 67
assessment 74
burns 86

checklist to aid assessment and management 71
management 76, 82–3
risk of violence among psychiatric inpatients 72
safety in the community 85
safety in outpatient settings 84
schizophrenia 70
terminology 70
warning signs 70
agnosias 12
agoraphobia 280
agranulocytosis 175
airway obstruction, causes of 36
alcohol misuse and dependence 102, 111, 137, 316
assessment 144
consumption levels 139
delirium 19
dependence 142
disabilities, alcohol-related 140–1
during pregnancy 241
intoxication 146, 316
units of alcohol 138
and violence 69
withdrawal 147, 172, 195
alcoholic hallucinosis 141
amenorrhoea 248
amisulpride 55
amphetamine and related substances 162–3
analgesia 242, 245
anhydrous glucose 43
anticholinergic drugs 174
anticonvulsant drugs 82, 163, 241
antidepressants 31, 245
atypical complicated grief 224
depressive and dysphoric symptomatology 62
eating disorders 257
and hyponatraemia 176
panic disorder 280
phobic disorders 280
post-traumatic stress disorder 282

postnatal puerperal depression 235
psychological consequences of surgery 218
puerperal psychosis 238
and suicide 128–9
violence 83
see also tricyclic antidepressants
antihypertensive drugs 197
antimuscarinic drugs 25, 174
antipsychotic drugs 163, 195
acute dystonia 174
acute pyschoses 54
amenorrhoea 248
morbid jealousy 93–4
oculogyric crisis 25
old-age psychiatry 268
pregnancy and childbirth 241
puerperal psychosis 238
violence 76, 82
antisocial personality 312
anxiety and depressive disorder, mixed 280
anxiety disorders 58–60, 276–9, 279
anxiolytic drugs 268
appearance 8
apraxia 12
aripiprazole 55
arrested or incomplete development of mind 296
assertive community treatment 283–92, 285
Assertive Outreach Services 285
assessment of emergencies 1
emergency referrals 2
information sources 5
interview arrangements 4
interview process 6
investigations 13
major emergencies 5
mental state examination 8–9
Mini-Mental State Examination 10–11
physical examination 12
telephone referrals 3

telepsychiatry 14
asthma, acute severe 45
attention 9 10
Australia 288
Austria 121
automatic obedience 64

B

bag-mask ventilation by two
    people 39
barbiturates 158
battered women syndrome
    90
Beck's Suicide Intent Scale
    132
beds, lack of to admit
    patients 316
behaviour 8
behavioural disturbance
    in siblings 234
behavioural interventions
    and violence 77
beliefs, abnormal 9
benzatropine 25, 31, 174
benzodiazepines 245
    anxiety and panic
        disorders 60–1
    atypical complicated grief
        224
    delirium 21
    oculogyric crisis 24
    paradoxical reactions
        181
    poisoning 29
    pregnancy and childbirth
        241
    psychological
        consequences of
        surgery 218
    referral to medical
        services 172
    sedatives and hypnotics
        158, 158
    substance abuse 171
    violence 76, 82
bereavement 222
best interests 307
beta-blockers 29, 83, 197
biochemical causes of
    puerperal psychosis 237
biological factors and
    violence 69
bite wounds, human 49
blood count, full 53
blood tests 13, 53
body dysmorphic disorders
    and other associated
    concepts 210
body image disorders 12
borderline personality 312
boredom 314
Bournewood gap 307

bradycardia resuscitation
    algorithm 40
brain imaging 53
brain syndrome 196
breaking bad news 220–1
breastfeeding 241
bromocriptine 26, 245
buprenorphine 152, 154,
    242
burns 86

C

caffeine 164
CAGE questionnaire 144
Canada 90
cancer 140
cannabinoids 156–7
capacity, assessment of
    305
capacity, emergency
    assessment of 136
carbamazepine 24, 55, 82
carbon monoxide 29
cardiomyopathy 175
cardiorespiratory support
    153
cardiovascular system
    changes 140
care programme approach
    125
Care Order 251
catalepsy 64
catatonic patients 64
central nervous system
    disorders 20
cerebral tumours 200
child abduction 89
Child Abduction Act 1984
    89
child abuse 254–5
child sexual abuse,
    consequences for adult
    functioning of 89
Children Act 1989 251
children and adolescents
    249–58
    assessment 250
    child abuse 254–5
    Children Act 1989 251
    eating disorders 256
    minors and consent 258
    non-accidental injury 88
    psychotropic medication-
        related complications
        257
    safety issues 251
    self-harm 252
    transition to adult services
        257
chin lift 37
chloral hydrate derivatives
    158

chloroquine 24
chlorpromazine 55
Cipralex 128
Cipramil 128
circumstances relating to
    suicide 132
cisplatin 24, 25
citalopram 128, 129
Class A drugs 150
Class B drugs 150
Class C drugs 150
clinical features and
    violence 75
clomipramine 179, 280,
    281
clonazepam 82
clonidine 153
clouding of consciousness
    212
clozapine 175
cocaine 111, 160–1
Code of Practice 113, 302,
    307
cognitive behaviour therapy
    104
cognitive state 9
cognitive symptoms and
    acute psychoses 52
coma 46, 56, 146
combination treatment
    80
comforting offences 89
Committee on Safety of
    Medicines 128, 128–9,
    175, 176
Community Rehabilitation
    Order 320, 325, 326
concentration 10
confabulation 196
confusional states, acute
    194–5, 196
conscious and ambulant
    persons 146
consent to treatment 258,
    303
conversion disorders 204,
    207
Coroners' Courts 329
countertransference 310
court diversion schemes
    320
Court of Protection 302,
    306
Court-Appointed Deputies
    213, 306
Couvade syndrome 240
crime 141
    see also violence and
        aggression
crisis resolution 288–9
Crown Court 319–30
cyanide 29
cyproheptadine 176

D

danazol 245
dangerousness 70
dantrolene 22
deliberate self-harm and
  suicide 115, 192, 252
  assessment form 134
  capacity, emergency
    assessment of 136
  deliberate self-harm
    116
  discharge 135
  National Confidential
    Enquiry into Suicide
    and Homicide in the
    UK 124–5
  non-fatal deliberate
    self-harm, management/
    prognosis/prevention
    of 118
  referral pathways 130
  repeated self-mutilation
    116
  suicidal intent, assessment
    of and risk of
    repetition 118
  suicide, assessment and
    management of
    132–3
  suicide, association of
    with antidepressant
    therapy 128–9
  suicide, association of
    with general practice
    consultation 122
  suicide, association of
    with physical disorders
    120
  suicide, association of
    with psychiatric
    disorders 119
  suicide, association of
    with psychiatric
    hospitalization 121
delirium 18–21, 194–5
delusions of passivity 53
delusions of thought
  interference 53
dementia 18, 196
demographic factors and
  violence 75
demographic risk factors
  for suicide 119
demoralization 314
denial of illness 314
Denmark 121
dependency 314
Depixol 83
depression 281
  postnatal puerperal 232–5
  see also post-partum
    maternity 'blues'

depressive and anxiety
  disorder, mixed 280
depressive disorders 229,
  278
depressive episodes 18,
  119
depressive symptomatology
  62
desipramine 160
Detained Resident status
  307
dexamfetamine sulphate
  162
dextrose 46
diabetic ketoacidosis and
  other diabetic
  emergencies 46–7
diagnostic factors and
  violence 75
diazepam 31, 88
  acute dystonia 174
  acute pyschoses 55
  violence 76
difficult patients and difficult
  situations 309–18
  management 312
  particular situations 316
  psychodynamic aspects of
    management 312
  understanding psychody-
    namics of being
    mentally disordered
    314
digoxin 197
dimethyltryptamine 166
disabilities, alcohol-related
  140–1
disaster see abuse, violence
  and disaster, victims of
discharge from hospital
  against medical advice
  316
dissociative disorders 204,
  207
diuretics 31, 245
diversion 320
Domestic Violence, Crime
  and Victims Act 2004
  321
dopamine agonists 26
dosulepin (previously
  dothiepin) 129
driving 272
drug abuse 111, 149
drug dependence 149
drug factors and violence
  69
drugs and delirium 19
drugs, negligent use of
  330
Duphaston 245
dydrogesterone 245
dysphoric mania 119

dysphoric symptomatology
  62
dystonia, acute 174
dystonic reactions, general
  22

E

early diversion 320
early intervention services
  290–2
eating disorders 256, 257
eating/drinking,
  withdrawal/refusal of
  64
echolalia 64
echopraxia 64
ecstasy (MDMA) 29, 166,
  167, 168
Edinburgh Postnatal
  Depression Scale 233
Effexor 128
egocentricity, increased
  314
elder abuse 92
electrocardiogram 53
electroconvulsive therapy:
  catatonia 65
  depressive and dysphoric
    symptomatology 62
  puerperal psychosis 238
electroencephalography 13,
  53
electrolytes 53
emotional immaturity 234
encephalitis 201
endocrine causes of organic
  anxiety disorder 59
endocrine disorders
  19–20, 63, 195
endocrinopathies 56
environment factors and
  violence 71, 69
environmental interventions
  and violence 77
envy 93–4
epilepsy, psychiatric aspects
  of 200
erotomania (de Cléram-
  bault's syndrome) 95
escitalopram 128
ethnic minorities 125
euphoric mania 119
Europe 283–92
euthymia 119
evening primrose oil 245
events, interpretations of 9
experiences, abnormal 9
expert evidence for court
  324–5
explaining the relationship
  of mental illness to
  offending 326

F

factitious disorder 207
factitious psychosis 186–7
failure to take patients
    seriously 314
false confessions 322
family factors and violence
    69
Faverin 128
fetal alcohol syndrome
    241
filicide 88
fitness to be interviewed by
    police 321
fitness to plead 321
fitness to remain in police
    custody 321
flumazenil 80, 82, 270
fluoxetine 128, 129
flupenthixol 83
fluvoxamine 128
forensic psychiatry 319–30
    expert evidence for court
        324–5
    police and court liaison
        320–2, 326–7
    prison psychiatry 328–9
forensic treatment orders
    for mentally abnormal
    offenders 298–9

G

gastrointestinal disorders
    140
general hospital medical
    wards 191–213
    assessment 212
    body dysmorphic
        disorders and other
        associated concepts
        210
    cerebral tumours 200
    common emergencies
        192
    dissociative and
        conversion disorders
        204
    epidemiology 192
    epilepsy 200
    HIV/AIDS 201
    Huntington's disease
        (chorea) 200
    hypochondriacal disorder
        204
    management 209
    medically unexplained
        symptoms 208
    memory disturbance 196
    meningitis, encephalitis
        and subarachnoid
        haemorrhages 201

mood disorder 197
multiple sclerosis 201
neurological symptoms,
    psychological reactions
    to 201
neurology 198–9
neurosyphilis 201
organic mental disorder/
    confusional states/
    delirium, acute
    194–5
Parkinsonism 201
patients taking leave
    against medical advice
    213
physical illness, factors
    influencing response
    to 208
physical and psychiatric
    illness, interaction
    between 202–3
prevention 192
somatization disorder
    206
uncooperative patient
    212
general medical conditions
    and violence 74
generalized anxiety
    disorders 278
    psychological features
        278
    somatic clinical features
        279
Gillick competence 258
glucagon 46
grief, atypical complicated
    224–5
gynaecology see obstetrics
    and gynaecology

H

haematological
    complications 140
hallucinogens 166–8
haloperidol 21, 76, 82, 195
hashish 156
head injury 198, 199, 327
head tilt 37
heparin 46
hepatic damage 140
histrionic personality 312
HIV/AIDS 201
Home Office 320
home treatment teams,
    intensive 288–9
homelessness, loneliness
    and isolation 109, 125
    loneliness 111
    management 112, 113
    prevalences and factors
        associated with 110

psychiatric disorders 111
homicide 128–9
hormonal causes of
    puerperal psychosis 237
hospital admission,
    demands for 316
Hospital Order 320, 321
Huntington's disease
    (chorea) 200
hyperemesis gravidarum
    (morning sickness) 228
hyperglycaemic hyperosmo-
    lar non-ketotic coma 46
hyperlactataemia 47
hypnotics 158–9
hypochondriacal disorder
    204
hypoglycaemic coma 46
hyponatraemia and
    antidepressants 176
hysterectomy 248

I

illicit drug screen 13
imipramine 179
immediate recall, good 196
immobility 64
Independent Mental
    Capacity Advocate 306
infection and organic
    mental disorder/
    confusional states/
    delirium 194
infertility 228
inflammatory disorders 59
informal inpatient 316
information, lack of 314
information sources 5
insight 9
insulin 46
Intensive Case Management
    Teams 283–92
Intensive Psychiatric
    Community Care
    283–92
interventions, emergency
    16
interview arrangements 4
interview process 6
intimate partner abuse 90
intoxication 59
intra familial causes of
    violence 68
intracranial causes of
    delirium 19
intracranial causes of
    organic anxiety disorder
    59
intracranial causes of organic
    mood disorders 63
investigations 13

isolation see homelessness, loneliness and isolation

J

Japan 233
jaw thrust 37

K

ketamine 166, 167
Korsakov's (Korsakoff's) psychosis 196

L

lactational psychoses 229
language functions 10
laryngeal mask airway insertion 39
Lasting Powers of Attorney 306
learning disabilities 259–61
  management 261
  medical problems, common 260
  mild 327
  potential problems 260
  presentation 260
levodopa 24
lithium 24, 31, 245
  acute pyschoses 55
  pregnancy and childbirth 241
  violence 83
liver function tests 53
Local Authorities 307
lofexidine 154
loneliness see homelessness, loneliness and isolation
lorazepam 31
  acute pyschoses 54
  catatonia 65
  old-age psychiatry 270
  violence 76, 82
lucid intervals 236
Lund and Browder charts 86
Lustral 128
lysergic acid diethylamine (LSD) 166

M

Magistrates Court 320
magnesium 43
majijuana 156
major emergencies 5
maladaptive psychological reactions to illness 202
malingering 207

management of
  emergencies 15
  asthma, acute severe 15
  delirium 18–21
  diabetic ketoacidosis and other diabetic emergencies 46–7
  dystonic reactions, general 22
  emergency interventions 16
  human bite wounds 49
  needlestick injuries 49
  neuroleptic malignant syndrome 26
  notifiable diseases 48
  oculogyric crisis 24–5
  poisoning 28–31
  resuscitation 34
  Wernicke's encephalo-pathy 42–3
mania 238
manipulative offences 89
manipulative patient 314–15
manner 8
matricide 88
mebeverene 154
medical advice, acting against 316
medical drugs leading to psychiatric complications 203
medically unexplained symptoms 188, 208
medication 63
  demands for 316
  old-age psychiatry 268
  to be avoided while taking monoamine oxidase inhibitors 178–9
medium secure units 321
memory 9
  disturbance 196
  for past events, poor 196
meningitis 201
menopause 247
Mental Capacity Act 2005 213, 304, 305, 306
  Code of Practice 307
  ill treatment or neglect of person who lacks capacity 306
mental disorder 296
mental fitness, issues of 329
Mental Health Act 1983/2007 149, 294, 296–300, 297, 301
  acting against medical advice 316
  aggression and violence 82

alcohol dependency 316
beds, lack of to admit patients 316
*the 'four stage' as introduced in Mental Health Bill 2006 308
consent to treatment 303
detention on general medical or surgical ward 304
emergency assessment of capacity 136
expert evidence for court 320
fitness to remain in police custody 321
forensic psychiatry 319–30
homelessness 113
and Mental Capacity Act 2005 307
and mental health review tribunals 301
old-age psychiatry 270
patients' rights 303
personality disorder 326
poisoning 28
post-traumatic stress disorder 100
prison psychiatry 328–9, 329
psychiatric opinions in Civil Law 329
puerperal psychosis 237
taking leave against medical advice 202–3
Mental Health Act Commission 302, 303
Mental Health Bill 2006 307, 308
Mental Health Commissioners 113
mental health legislation 293–308
  consent to treatment 303
  Court of Protection 302
  Mental Health Act Commission 302
  see also Mental Capacity Act 2005; Mental Health Act
Mental Health Review Tribunals 301, 303, 320
mental illness 296
mental impairment 296
mental retardation 296
mental state examination 8–9, 144
Mental Welfare Commission 301
mescaline 166
metabolic disorders 19–20

metabolic disturbance 195
methadone 152, 153, 154
methylphenidate
    hydrochloride 102, 257
metoclopramide 24, 25, 154
mild mental retardation
    296
Mini-Mental State
    Examination 10–11
mirtazapine 128
miscarriage, recurrent 228
missed contact 124
Misuse of Drugs Act 1971
    150
Modernization Teams
    283–92
monitoring schedule 82
monoamine oxidase
    inhibitors 178, 235, 280
foods to be avoided while
    taking monoamine
    oxidase inhibitors 178
mood 8
    changes 141
    disorder 197
    symptoms and acute
        psychoses 52
morbid jealousy (Othello
    syndrome) 93
mother–infant relationship
    234, 244
motility 8
mouth-to-mask ventilation
    38
multiple sclerosis 201
Munchausen syndrome by
    proxy 186
Munchausen syndrome
    (hospital addiction
    syndrome) 186–7
muscle disorders 140–1
muscle rigidity 64
mutism 64
myocarditis 175
myxoedema coma 56

N

naloxone 153
National Assembly 307
National Confidential
    Enquiry into Suicide
    and Homicide in the UK
    124–5
needle exchange
    programmes 153
needlestick injuries 49
negative symptoms and
    acute psychoses 52
negativism 64
nerve disorders 140–1
neuroimaging 13
neuroleptic drugs 82, 248

neuroleptic malignant
    syndrome 26
neurological disorder 195
neurological symptoms,
    psychological reactions
    to 201
neurology, psychiatric
    aspects of 198–9
neuropsychological tests 13
neuroses 199
neurosyphilis 201
neurotic and stress-related
    disorders 276–82
    anxiety and depressive
        disorder, mixed 280
    anxiety disorders 276–9
    anxiety, disorders
        presenting primarily
        with symptoms of 279
    depression 281
    factors associated with
        development of 276
    frequency of neurotic
        conditions 276–7
    generalized anxiety and
        depressive disorders
        278
    generalized anxiety
        disorder, psychological
        features of 278
    generalized anxiety
        disorder, somatic
        clinical features of 279
    neurosis, concept of 276
    obsessive-compulsive
        disorder 281
    panic disorder 280, 281
    phobias and behavioural
        learning theory 281
    phobic disorders 280, 281
    post-traumatic stress
        disorder 282
New Zealand 122, 132, 233
nicotinamide 43
nicotinic acid deficiencies 43
nifedipine 24
non-accidental injury of
    children 88
non-compliance with
    treatment 124
non-opiate medication 154
non-psychiatric causes of
    violence 68
non-steroidal anti-
    inflammatory drugs 31
notifiable diseases 48

O

obsessive-compulsive
    disorder 281
obstetrics and gynaecology
    227–48

alcohol during pregnancy
    241
amenorrhoea 248
Couvade syndrome 240
fetal alcohol syndrome
    241
hysterectomy 248
menopause 247
mother–infantrelationship
    244
opioid dependence and
    withdrawal in
    pregnancy 242
oral contraception 244
perinatal psychiatry 228
post-partum maternity
    'blues' 230
postnatal puerperal
    depression 232–5
pregnancy termination
    244–5
premenstrual syndrome
    245–7
psychotropic drugs during
    pregnancy and
    lactation 240–1
puerperal psychosis
    236–8
puerperal women, role
    of trainee in initial
    assessment of 239
sterilization 245
stillbirth 244
oculogyric crisis 24–5
oestrogen 245, 247
olanzapine 55, 268
old-age psychiatry 263–72
    accident and emergency
        departments 266, 271
    driving 272
    general managment issues
        272
    medication 268
    presentation of psychiatric
        disorders 264
oncology see surgery,
    radiotherapy, oncology
    and terminal illness
opiates 29
    withdrawal, management
        of 154
opioids 152–3
    dependence and
        withdrawal in
        pregnancy 242
    replacement 154
    withdrawal 172
oppositionism/gegenhalten
    64
oral contraception 244, 245
organ failure 19
organic causes of catatonia
    64

organic mental disorders 194–5, 202
organic reaction psychosis 196
organophosphate insecticides 29
orientation in place 10
orientation in time 10
oropharyngeal airway insertion 38
overdependent personalities 234
overdose of medication 316
oxycodone 152
oxygen 45, 47

P

Pabrinex 43
pandemic infection outbreaks 102
panic disorders 58–60, 280, 281
paracetamol 29
paranoid patient 312
paraquat 29
Parkinsonism 201
Parole Board 328–9
paroxetine 128
past history and violence 75
pathological lying 186–7
patient and physical illness 208
patient and violence 71
patient–therapist relationship variable 78
pentazocine 152
perinatal psychiatry 228
personal social support, absence of 233
personality change 198
personality disorder 326
phencyclidine 166, 167
phenelzine 280
phenothiazines 31
phenytoin 241
phobias and behavioural learning theory 281
phobic disorders 280, 281
physical complaints, physical conditions presenting with 202
physical complaints, psychiatric conditions presenting with 202
physical conditions and mood disorder 197
physical dependence (addiction) 149
physical effects of hallucinogens 167

physical examination 12, 144
physical illness, factors influencing response to 208
physical morbidity and alcohol-related disabilities 140–1
physical and psychiatric illness, interaction between 202–3
physical symptoms and cannabinoids 156
poisoning 28–31
police and court liaison 320–2, 326–7
police diversion schemes 320
police involvement following violence 316
positive psychotic symptoms 212
positive symptoms and acute psychoses 52
post-discharge follow-up 125
post-partum maternity 'blues' 229, 230
post-partum psychiatric disorders 228–9
post-traumatic stress disorder 95, 100–4, 282
postnatal depression 229
postnatal puerperal depression 232–5
posturing 64
potential victims and violence 71
Powers of Attorney 213
pregnancy 228
  termination 244–5
  test 53
premenstrual syndrome 245–7
previous psychiatric history of depressive disorder 233
primary care 273–83
  epidemiology 274
  range of cases compared to psychiatric practice 275
  safety considerations 282
  see also neurotic and stress-related disorders
Primary Care Trusts 307
Prison Medical Officers 328–9
prison psychiatry 328–9
prochlorperazine 31

procyclidine 25, 80, 82, 174, 270
prodromal period 236
progesterones 245
projective identification 310
propranolol 83
Protection from Harassment Act 1997 95
Prozac 128
psilocybin 166
psychiatric assessment and poisoning 28
psychiatric causes of violence 74, 68
psychiatric damage, issues of 329–30
psychiatric disorders and violence 69
psychiatric drugs leading to medical complications 203
psychiatric (functional) causes of catatonia 64
psychiatric morbidity and alcohol-related disabilities 141
psychiatric negligence 330
psychiatric opinions in civil law 329–30
psychiatric risk factors for suicide 119
psychoactive substance misuse 59, 63, 149
  amphetamine and related substances 162–3
  caffeine 164
  cannabinoids 156–7
  cocaine 160–1
  examination 171
  hallucinogens 166–8
  history-taking relevant to 171
  investigations 172
  Misuse of Drugs Act 1971 150
  opiate withdrawal, management of 154
  opioids 152–3
  referral to medical services 172
  referral to specialist substance misuse services 172
  sedatives and hypnotics 158–9
  solvents, volatile 170
psychodynamic aspects of management of psychiatric emergencies 312
psychodynamic factors and puerperal psychosis 237

psychodynamic models and violence 69
psychological dependence (habituation) 149
psychological effects and cannabinoids 156–7
psychological effects of hallucinogens 168
psychological factors and violence 75
psychological models and violence 69
psychological symptoms and premenstrual syndrome 247
psychopathic disorder 300
psychoses, acute 52–4
psychosexual disorders 141
psychosis 111
puerperal 236–8
psychosocial risk factors for suicide 119
psychosomatic disease 202
psychostimulants 162
psychotherapeutic approach, potential artificial nature of 314
psychotic depression 238
psychotic offences 89
psychotropic drug actions, emergencies related to 173–81
benzodiazepines, paradoxical reactions to 181
clozapine 175
dystonia, acute 174
hyponatraemia and antidepressants 176
monoamine oxidase inhibitors 178
serotonin syndrome 176
psychotropic drugs 241
psychotropic medication-related complications 257
Public Guardian 306
puerperal psychiatric disorders 229
puerperal psychosis 229, 236–8
puerperal women, role of trainee in initial assessment of 239
pyridoxine 245

Q

quetiapine 55, 76

R

radiotherapy see surgery, radiotherapy, oncology and terminal illness
random blood glucose 53
rape of men 98–9
rape of women 96–7
recall 10
referral:
emergency 2
pathways 130
registration 10
rehydration 46
relatives, demanding 316
relaxation therapy 245
repetitive transcranial magnetic stimulation 62
resperpine 24
restraint 307
Restriction Order 320
resuscitation 34
adult advanced cardiac arrest life support algorithm 35
airway obstruction, causes of 36
algorithm for resuscitation of hospital inpatients 34
bag-mask ventilation by two people 39
bradycardia resuscitation algorithm 40
equipment, emergency 80, 82, 270
head tilt and chin lift 37
jaw thrust 37
laryngeal mask airway insertion 39
mouth-to-mask ventilation 38
oropharyngeal airway insertion 38
tachycardia resuscitation algorithm 41
rigid, obsessional personalities 234
risk 70, 133
management plan 76
risperidone 55, 268
rivalry 93–4
routine postoperative screening 217

S

safety considerations in primary care 282
safety issues with children and adolescents 251
salbutamol 45

salicylate (aspirin) 29
schizophrenia 194–5
acute psychoses 53
aggression and violence 70
delirium 18
homelessness 111
perinatal psychiatry 229
puerperal psychosis 238
suicide 119
schizophreniform psychosis 199
sedation 163
guidelines for accident and emergency departments 79
sedatives 158–9, 268
selective serotonin re-uptake inhibitors:
children and adolescents 128
deliberate self-harm and suicide 128–9, 129
hyponatraemia 176
obsessive-compulsive disorder 281
panic disorder 280
poisoning 31
post-traumatic stress disorder 104
premenstrual syndrome 245
serotonin syndrome 176
violence 83
self-report 133
serotonin syndrome 176
Seroxat 128
sertraline 128
severe mental impairment 296
sexual assault of men 98–9
sexual assault of women 96–7
Singapore 233
social environment and physical illness 208
social models and violence 69
social morbidity and alcohol-related disabilities 141
social phobia 280
sodium bicarbonate 31
solvents, volatile 170
somatization disorder 206
somatoform disorders 207
Special Hospitals 320–1

specific phobias 280
speech 8
spironolactone 245
splitting 310
squinve house 90–1
staff and law and violence 72
stalking 95
sterilization 245
steroids 45, 197
stigma 314
stillbirth 244
stress reaction, acute 106
stress-related disorders
  see neurotic and
  stress-related disorders
  276–82
stressful life events 233
stressful work
  environments 102
stupor 64
subarachnoid haemorrhages 201
substance misuse 111, 192, 326
  disorders 74, 119
  see also psychoactive
    substance misuse
suicidal thoughts 111
suicide 330
  attempted 330
  inpatient 124
  rate 236
  risk in prison 328–9
  threatening by
    telephone calls 316
  see also deliberate
    self-harm and suicide
Supervision Order 251, 321
Supreme Court 302
surgery, radiotherapy,
  oncology and terminal
  illness 215–25
  bereavement 222
  dying, management of 220
  grief, atypical complicated 224–5
  surgery, psychological
    consequences of 216–17

symptoms and syndromes
  presenting as
  emergencies 51
  lethargy and panic,
    disorders presenting
    with 58–60
  catatonic patients 64
  depressive and dysphoric
    symptomatology 62
  endocrinopathies 56
  psychoses, acute 52–4
systemic disorders 59, 63
systemic infections 20

T

tachycardia resuscitation
  algorithm 41
taking leave against medical
  advice 213
telephone referrals 3
telepsychiatry 14
terminal illness see surgery,
  radiotherapy, oncology
  and terminal illness
terror 314
terrorism 102
thiamine replacement 43
third-person auditory
  hallucinations 53
thought 8
  disorder 53
  echo 53
thyrotoxic storm 56
toxicity with many
  prescribed drugs 19
Training in Community
  Living 283–92
tranquillization, rapid 76
transference 310
tranylcypromine 179
trauma 140
tricyclic antidepressants
  31, 129, 179
  cocaine 160
  oculogyric crisis 24
  old-age psychiatry 268
  pregnancy and childbirth 241
trifluoperazine 31

U

unco-operative patient 213
United Arab Emirates 233
United States 90–1, 110,
  111, 241, 283–92, 285
urea 53
urine acidification 163
urine drug screen 53

V

Valium 88
valproate 55, 82
venlafaxine 128, 129
verbal approach to violence
  77
verbigeration 64
violence 70
  and acute intoxication 146
  cognitive 74
  emotional 74
  police involvement
    following 316
  psychodynamic
    formulation 310–11
  staff role in precipitating 310
  see also abuse, violence
    and disaster, victims
    of; aggression and
    violence
vitamin B 43
vitamin C 43
vitamin deficiency 59, 195
vulnerability factors 102

W

waxy flexibility 64
Wernicke's encephalopathy
  42–3

Z

Zispin 128
zolpidem 154
zopiclone 154
zuclopentixol acetate 76